Abdalla Bowirrat
Awni Youssef
Mustafa Yassin

Cerebral Subcortical infarcts with Leukoencephalopathy

Abdalla Bowirrat
Awni Youssef
Mustafa Yassin

Cerebral Subcortical infarcts with Leukoencephalopathy

LAP LAMBERT Academic Publishing

Impressum / Imprint

Bibliografische Information der Deutschen Nationalbibliothek: Die Deutsche Nationalbibliothek verzeichnet diese Publikation in der Deutschen Nationalbibliografie; detaillierte bibliografische Daten sind im Internet über http://dnb.d-nb.de abrufbar.

Alle in diesem Buch genannten Marken und Produktnamen unterliegen warenzeichen-, marken- oder patentrechtlichem Schutz bzw. sind Warenzeichen oder eingetragene Warenzeichen der jeweiligen Inhaber. Die Wiedergabe von Marken, Produktnamen, Gebrauchsnamen, Handelsnamen, Warenbezeichnungen u.s.w. in diesem Werk berechtigt auch ohne besondere Kennzeichnung nicht zu der Annahme, dass solche Namen im Sinne der Warenzeichen- und Markenschutzgesetzgebung als frei zu betrachten wären und daher von jedermann benutzt werden dürften.

Bibliographic information published by the Deutsche Nationalbibliothek: The Deutsche Nationalbibliothek lists this publication in the Deutsche Nationalbibliografie; detailed bibliographic data are available in the Internet at http://dnb.d-nb.de.

Any brand names and product names mentioned in this book are subject to trademark, brand or patent protection and are trademarks or registered trademarks of their respective holders. The use of brand names, product names, common names, trade names, product descriptions etc. even without a particular marking in this work is in no way to be construed to mean that such names may be regarded as unrestricted in respect of trademark and brand protection legislation and could thus be used by anyone.

Coverbild / Cover image: www.ingimage.com

Verlag / Publisher:
LAP LAMBERT Academic Publishing
ist ein Imprint der / is a trademark of
OmniScriptum GmbH & Co. KG
Heinrich-Böcking-Str. 6-8, 66121 Saarbrücken, Deutschland / Germany
Email: info@lap-publishing.com

Herstellung: siehe letzte Seite /
Printed at: see last page
ISBN: 978-3-659-64903-5

Cerebral Autosomal Dominant Arteriopathy with Subcortical Infarcts and Leukoencephalopathy (CADASIL)

Prof. Dr. Bowirrat Abdalla M.D., Ph.D.
Prof. of Clinical Neuroscience and Population Genetics – Director of Research Center, EMMS Nazareth Hospital,   Faculty of Medicine in the Galilee, Bar Ilan University.
Tel: +972 4635-6133; Mobile: +972 54-669-3763
 Email: Prof.Bowirrat@yahoo.com;_bowirrat@Gmail.com

Co-Authors

Dr. Awni youssef M.D., MPH.
Head of Medical Consulting Center, Nazareath Towers, General Medical Services " sheruti briut clalit" Email: zaawniyo@clalit.org.il;
Mobile: +972-54-5242723.

Dr. Yassin Mustafa, specialist in orthopedic surgery, Rabin Medical Center, Campus Hasharon, Petah Tikva, Israel.
Email: mustafay@clalit.org.il
Mobile: +972-50- 5247811

Table of content

Overview of CADASIL:

Summary

Cerebral autosomal dominant arteriopathy with subcortical infarcts and leukoencephalopathy (CADASIL, OMIM #125310) is a rare mid-adult onset monogenic form of hereditary cerebral microangiopathy, caused by mutations in the NOTCH3 gene which lead to abnormal extracellular matrix accumulation of granular osmiophilic material (GOM) in the vicinity of vascular smooth muscle cells (VSMCs) causing degeneration and loss of VSMCs in small arteries and arterioles. Clinically the syndrome is manifested as migraine with aura, recurrent subcortical ischaemic events or strokes, subcortical vascular dementia and mood disorders. Strokes are typically ischemic, while hemorrhagic events have been only sporadically described. Diagnosis of CADASIL is established on the basis of results of genetic testing; skin biopsy and MRI. However, a genetic test is the gold standard to confirm the diagnosis and to identify a mutation in the underlying gene NOTCH3, which is caused by at least 170 mutations in the NOTCH3 gene at locus 19p13.1–13.26.

Pathological test used to identify the GOM deposition around VSMCs examined by electron microscopy in skin biopsies is considered a specific diagnostic tool for CADASIL. In addition, imaging abnormalities in CADASIL evolve as the disease progresses: Typical MRI findings are T2 weighted hyperintensities in white matter and the capsula externa, Subcortical lacunar lesions and cerebral microbleeds are seen.

The Pathogenesis of Cerebral Autosomal Dominant Arteriopathy with Subcortical Infarcts and Leukoencephalopathy (CADASIL, OMIM #125310)

Summary

Cerebral autosomal dominant arteriopathy with subcortical infarcts and leukoencephalopathy (CADASIL, OMIM #125310) is a rare hereditary systemic vasculopathy and an example of pleiotropism i.e. single gene effects on multiple phenotypic traits. CADASIL is the most common monogenic form of hereditary cerebral microangiopathy disorder manifesting usually in early adulthood which cause a highly stereotyped mutations within the extracellular domain of the NOTCH3 gene. NOTCH3 mutations within the receptor extracellular domain, lead to abnormal extracellular matrix accumulation of granular osmiophilic material (GOM) in the close vicinity of vascular smooth muscle cells (VSMCs) and around small caliber arteries and arterioles, eventually leading to a progressive loss of VSMCs. In the brain, degeneration of smooth muscle cells in small arteries results in an impaired cerebral blood flow, arteriolar stenosis and lacunar infarcts, mainly in cerebral white matter and deep gray matter. Affected individuals exhibit a variety of symptoms, and clinical presentation of CADASIL varies even among and within families. The disease is characterized by six main symptoms: migraine with aura, subcortical ischemic events, mood disturbances, apathy, cognitive impairment and subcortical dementia. Usually, at the age of 30–50, patients begin to suffer from recurrent transient ischaemic attacks (TIAs) or ischaemic strokes due to subcortical lacunar infarcts. These will eventually lead to a progressive cognitive decline, psychiatric disorders, and to a subcortical type of vascular dementia. Strokes are typically ischemic, while hemorrhagic events have been only sporadically described. However, cerebral microbleeds have been found in 31-69% of CADASIL patients. CADASIL phenotype is highly variable and although the full clinical-neuroimaging picture may be suggestive of the disease, three methods are usually needed to confirm the diagnosis of CADASIL: The genetic testing; skin biopsy and MRI. However, a genetic test remains the diagnostic gold standard to confirm the diagnosis and to identify a mutation in the underlying gene NOTCH3 encoding a transmembrane receptor protein, which is caused by at least 200 mutations in the NOTCH3 gene at locus 19p13.1–13.26. NOTCH3 mutations are usually assessed by restriction enzyme analysis of specific mutations or by sequence analysis; pathological test used to identify the GOM deposition around VSMCs examined by electron microscopy (EM) in skin biopsies is extremely helpful and considered a specific diagnostic tool for CADASIL. In addition, imaging abnormalities in CADASIL evolve as the disease progresses: Typical MRI findings are T2 weighted hyperintensities in white matter and the capsula externa, Subcortical lacunar lesions (SLLs) and Cerebral microbleeds are usually seen.

Candidate Biomarkers and CSF Profiles for Alzheimer's disease and CADASIL

<u>Summary</u>

To differentiate neurodegenerative disorder such as Alzheimer's disease (AD) from vascular dementia (VaD) is not a simple process, the procedure still roughly problematic in clinical practice, despite the widely used diagnostic criteria to differentiate between the two disorders. There are plethora of evidences that support the involvement of cerebrovascular dysfunction not only in vascular causes of cognitive deficits observed in vascular dementia, but also in the underpinning causes of cognitive deterioration of AD.

Cognitively patients, with AD, show sometimes mixed degrees of associated vascular lesions in 30-60% of AD cases. In opposition, cognitively patients, with VaD, may carry 40%-70% of AD pathology, consequently impeding diagnosis precision.

Therefore, to eliminate this bewilderment and discrepancies in the diagnosis between the AD and VaD, it is worthy to shed light firstly on a disease that is a microangiopathy and represents VaD with clear milestones and features as is the case of Cerebral Autosomal Dominant Arteriopathy with Subcortical Infarcts and Leukoencephalopathy (CADASIL). Studying CADASIL CSF biomarkers profile, will help in the differential diagnosis between both diseases sharing the coexisting neurodegeneration, furthermore, CADASIL is a dominantly inherited mid-adult life disorder causing ischemic strokes, which belongs to vasculopathies and symbolizes a genuine prototype of VaD that provides a valuable opportunity for studying its CSF biomarkers. Secondly, examining and evaluating the CSF biomarkers of AD compared to that of CADASIL.

The pathogenesis similarities between CADASIL and early onset AD affecting the small vessels of the brain have suggested plausible molecular mechanisms involved in vascular damage and their impact on brain function and also come from the fact that in both diseases genetic mutations occur. CADASIL mutations in NOTCH3 gene generate toxic protein aggregates (Granular Osmiophilic Material- GOM) in the surrounding area of Vascular Smooth Muscle Cells (VSMCs) causing degeneration in addition to loss of VSMCs in small arteries and arterioles of white matter regions of the brain that lead to dementia, similar to those attributed to mutant forms of the Amyloid Precursor proteins (APP) and presenilins genes who cause overproduction and accumulations of the toxic Aβ42 protein in the brain and collapse of Aβ42 clearance mechanisms in AD. Despite the presumed pathological similarities, substantial differences between the two phenomena may exist especially in the CSF neurochemical phenotypes [(CSF total tau (t-tau), β-amyloid protein 1-42, and phosphorylated tau (p-tau)]. In addition to the well known differences in neuroimaging between these diseases, our review comes to strengthen the importance and encourage the use of CSF biomarkers profile variations in the differential diagnosis between the neurodegenerative diseases in general and between AD and CADASIL in special.

Chapter 1 – Introduction to CADASIL

Background

Cerebral autosomal dominant arteriopathy with subcortical infarcts and leukoencephalopathy (CADASIL, OMIM #125310) is the most common form of hereditary cerebral angiopathy which affects mainly the brain, and is caused by over 170 different mutations in the *NOTCH3* gene at chromosome 19,[1-3] (Figure 1) which shows considerable genetic heterogeneity.[4,5]

The condition was first described more than 30 years ago in a Swedish family,[6] although the acronym CADASIL did not emerge until the early 1990s.[7] CADASIL is caused by mutations in NOTCH3 gene encoding a 280 kDa transmembrane receptor and is present in more than 90% of individuals. NOTCH3 is the only gene in which mutations are known to cause CADASIL.[8] The mutations cause progressive vascular smooth muscle cell (VSMC) degeneration, thickening and fibrosis of the vessel walls and accumulation of the Notch3 extracellular domain (N3ECD) on the VSMCs.[9,10]

Linked to mutations in the *NOTCH3* gene, CADASIL vasculopathy is considered the most common single gene form of hereditary cerebral angiopathy, caused by highly stereotyped mutations within the extracellular domain of the NOTCH3 receptor [Notch3 (ECD)] that result in an odd number of cysteine residues. The characteristic type of the mutations, which change the total number of cysteine residues within the epidermal growth factor-like repeats (EGFR), suggests that all mutations divide common mechanisms.[11,12]

Clinically, CADASIL, has various and different pathologies, is linked with cerebral infarcts in more than two third of cases, especially multi-lacunar infarcts engaging the subcortical white matter, deep gray matter nuclei, and brain stem, as well as progressive cognitive decline (subcortical dementia with pseudobulbar palsy and urinary incontinence) in half of cases which are the main clinical signs of CADASIL (Figure 2). Additional neurological manifestations include migraine with aura in 22%–64% of patients.[13, 14]

CADASIL is characterized by transient ischemic attacks or strokes observed in approximately 85% of symptomatic patients. A classic lacunar syndrome (small infarcts) occurs in at least two-thirds of affected patients while hemispheric strokes are much less common. It is worthy to note that ischemic strokes typically occur in the absence of traditional cardiovascular risk factors. Absence of hypertension or other known vascular risk factors is essential for the clinical diagnosis.[15-17]

The age of onset of CADASIL varies greatly, which also depends on the criterion used for the onset of the disease. At the age of 30–50, patients begin to suffer from recurrent transient ischaemic attacks (TIAs) or ischaemic strokes due to subcortical lacunar infarcts usually beginning after the age of 50. The age at the first ever stroke varies from approximately 25 to 70 years with a reported peak around 40-50 years of age and with great variation even within the same family,[18-20] and even between monozygotic twins.[21]

These cerebrovascular events will eventually lead to early cognitive impairment/dementia that progresses into frank dementia of subcortical type associated with pseudobulbar palsy and urinary incontinence later in life. Executive and organizing cognitive functions are impaired first, memory is affected late.[22] Cerebral microbleeds have been found in 31-69% of CADASIL patients.[23,24] Physiologically, cerebral blood volume and cerebral glucose utilization are significantly reduced.[25] Furthermore, cerebral vasoreactivity and fragility are impaired, consistent with the observed degeneration of vascular smooth muscle cells in small arteries and arterioles.[26]

Recurrent migraine attacks with aura (often atypical or isolated, seen in 30%-40% of individuals) sometimes accompanied with confusion, fever, meningitis or coma.

Progressive white matter degeneration are other features of the disease, in addition, affected individuals exhibit a variety of symptoms, including seizures, bipolar disorder, personality changes, mood disturbance, apathy, and premature death, commonly within 20-25 years after symptoms have occurred.[27-31]

The pathologic hallmark of CADASIL is electron-dense granules osmiophilic material (GOM), which contains extracellular domains of Notch3, in the media of arterioles that can often be identified by electron microscopic (EM) evaluation of skin biopsies. NOTCH3 mutations within the receptor extracellular domain leads to abnormal extracellular matrix accumulation of GOM and NOTCH3 extracellular domain around small caliber arteries and arterioles and eventual progressive loss of vascular smooth muscle cells.[9] CADASIL shows true dominancy and the vast majority of CADASIL mutations (95%) are missense mutations removing or inserting cysteine residues within 1–34 epidermal growth factor-like repeats in the *NOTCH3* protein. Small inframe deletions are observed and splice-site mutations in the *NOTCH3* gene encoding a transmembrane receptor are also seen, which invariably cause inframe deletions resulting in loss of cysteine residues.[32-36]

Indeed, six pathogenic deletions, one combined deletion and insertion (or two adjacent nucleotide substitutions), two duplications, and two splice-site mutations have been described. In addition to these common types of cysteine affecting CADASIL mutations, seven mutations not altering the number of cysteines have been reported. One of these mutations is a deletion which removes the amino acids between two cysteines, and the remainder is missense mutations leading to one amino acid substitution.[37, 38, 8, 32, 34]

Whether these substitutions are truly pathogenic mutations or merely variants is yet unclear. So far, only three reports of patients homozygous for pathogenic *NOTCH3* mutations have been published.[39-41]

In addition, two confirmed de novo mutations in CADASIL patients have been reported.[42, 43] Thus, either a cysteine residue is deleted or altered to another amino acid residue or, conversely, mutations of noncysteine residues lead to introduction of novel cysteine residues.[34] This results in an uneven number of cysteine residues in the

8

given domain, most likely modifying the tertiary structure of the protein.[32] At least three mechanisms mediate the pathogenic effects of *NOTCH3* mutation in CADASIL, i.e., loss of receptor function, gain of function, and neomorphic (eg, toxic) processes.

Mutations of *NOTCH3* characteristically lead to an epidermal growth factor-like repeat domain (six repeats in the normal domain) and an odd number of cysteine residues (either five or seven) through gain or loss of a residue.[8] Some researchers claim that no mutations leading to three cysteine residues or not involving a cysteine residue have ever been reported.[33, 44] However, it is not yet known whether these mutations primarily affect receptor trafficking, maturation, and/or signaling.[45]

The History of CADASIL

Historically, on the basis of thorough scrutiny of the literature, the first CADASIL family is now believed to have been reported in 1955 by Van Bogaert,[46, 47] who described two sisters with rapidly progressive subcortical encephalopathy of Binswanger's type.[48]

In 1977, Sourander and Walinder reported a Swedish family with a CADASIL mutation and multi-infarct dementia of autosomal-dominant inheritance, presenting with pyramidal, bulbar, and cerebellar symptoms, a relapsing course, and gradually evolving severe dementia.[6] In 2007, Low et al verified that the hereditary multi-infarct dementia in the Swedish family reported by Sourander and Walinder was erroneously attributed to CADASIL, and that the patients did not show the characteristic features of CADASIL on pathological examination.[49]

In Finland, the first family with CADASIL was identified and published as hereditary multi-infarct dementia in 1987.[50]

After the gene test became available, 15 new families comprising approximately 100 patients or presymptomatic carriers of the gene defect have been identified in Finland. Fourteen of the 15 families identified in Finland carry the same C475T transition mutation of the *NOTCH3* gene, which leads to substitution of the 133 arginine by cysteine (R133C).[51, 29, 50]

Information concerning the exact global incidence and prevalence of CADASIL is limited. In the west of Scotland, the prevalence of confirmed CADASIL cases in 2004 was 1.98/100,000 and the estimated prevalence based on pedigree information was 4.15/100,000.[50] In Finland, a similar prevalence has been estimated.[52, 53]

In 1993, Tournier-Lasserve et al operated linkage analysis to two extended distinct French families with CADASIL, and connected the disease to chromosome 19q12.14 a more recent study by Tikka et al investigated different pathogenic mutations in 34 patients in France, and demonstrated three novel point mutations (p.Cys67Ser, p.Cys251Tyr, and p.Tyr1069Cys) and a novel duplication (p.Glu434-Leu436dup). In this cohort, the congruence between *NOTCH3* mutations and deposition of granular osmiophilic material around vascular smooth muscle cells, which is the gold standard for confirmation of a diagnosis of CADASIL, was 100%.[1] In 2002, Markus et al performed a large genetic study of 48 British families and showed that most mutations of CADASIL were located in exon 4, followed by exons 3, 5, 6, 8, 18, and 22.[54]

Another study from a Dutch DNA diagnostic laboratory (44 Dutch and 22 foreign families) also found the mutation rate of CADASIL was highest in exon 4, followed by exon 3, 5, 6, 11, and 19.[55]

Thus, it is suggested that exons 3–6 should be screened first, and then exons 11 and 18–23. In fact, worldwide variations have been described, showing exon 3 to be the second most common mutation site in French, British, and German individuals,[34, 54, 56-57] while exon 11 frequently harbors mutations in affected Dutch individuals.[56]

Epidemiologically, the precise frequency and mortality rate of CADASIL worldwide is still unknown. The mean age of death has been reported to be 61 years after a mean disease duration of approximately 23 years.[19] Men tend to die earlier than women,[3] but mortality appears to be equally distributed between the genders, and the onset of clinical symptoms usually occurs in the fourth decade of life, with a mean age at presentation of 46.1 years.[58, 19]

Fewer than half of patients older than 60 years can walk without assistance and nearly 80% of patients are completely dependent immediately before death.[3]

However, the number of reported cases of CADASIL is gradually increasing as the clinical picture becomes more widely recognized and genetic testing becomes available. CADASIL occurs worldwide and has been reported in many ethnic groups. So far, most of the CADASIL patients have been found in Caucasian families, including France, Germany, the UK, Finland, Sweden, Italy, and the Netherlands.[14, 19, 51, 53, 56, 59-63]

Reports from North America are relatively sparse, despite the high level of academic activity in this region. In 2007, Bohlega et al.[64] studied three families from Arab countries (Saudi Arabia, Kuwait, and Yemen) containing 19 individuals affected by CADASIL. All *NOTCH3* exons were screened for mutations, which showed the presence of formerly described mutations in c.406C . T (p.Arg110 . Cys) in two families from the middle east (Saudi Arabia and Kuwait), and a c.475C . T (p.Arg133. Cys) mutation in the family from Yemen. The investigators concluded that CADASIL does occur in Arabs, with a clinical phenotype and genotype similar to that in other ethnic groups.

Overview of NOTCH Genes Subtypes (Figure 3)

In mammals, four Notch receptors (Notch 1–4) and five Notch ligands (Delta-like-1, -3, -4, Jagged-1, -2) have been described. An increasing body of evidence suggests that ligand-induced Notch signalling plays a pivotal role, both in various developmental contexts during embryonic development and also in adult tissues.[65-68]

The origin of the term 'Notch' stems from the observations of great genetics scientist Thomas Hunt Morgan,[69] who in 1917 published 'The Theory of the Gene' his paper described a mutant female drosophila fly with serrations at the ends of the wings, which he named 'Notch'. Another fly with a mutant wing shape he called 'Delta'. Decades later, it was observed that the mutant homologues of the fly genes that defects the exoskeleton also causes malformations of the endoskeleton in human.[69]

Currently, we comprehend the Notch pathway, of which Notch and Delta are parts, as a multifaceted intercellular signalling cascade system that is vital to natural development, one that has been preserved across animal species where the body plan contains tissues differentiated into muscles and nerves, that is, metazoans.

The Notch genes encode considerable cell surface transmembrane receptors whose role is to arbitrate fundamental cellular functions through direct cell–cell contact. The initiation of membrane-bound Notch by specific ligands results in proteolytic cleavage, by g-secretase activity, of the Notch intracellular domain (NICD) from the plasma membrane, and this protein directly translocates to the nucleus to play a role in the transcriptional regulation of target genes, where it converts downstream targets from transcriptional repressors to transcriptional activators.

In this mode the pathway influences cell destiny and lineage commitment through differentiation, proliferation and apoptosis in the procedures of neurogenesis, myogenesis, angiogenesis, haematopoiesis and epithelial–mesenchymal transition. A cornerstone role of the pathway is in the developmental integrity of somitogenesis.

Somites are paired blocks of tissue that form sequentially from the presomitic mesoderm (PSM) either side of the notochord in a rostrocaudal direction. Finally they differentiate into vertebrae, ribs, muscles, tendons and ligaments.

Germline mutations in Notch pathway genes give rise to a array of syndromes which, presently, can be clustered into: (1) The spondylocostal dysostosis (SCD); (2) Alagille syndrome (ALGS), NOTCH1-related congenital heart disease (CHD) and CADASIL; (3) Hajdu–Cheney syndrome (HJCYS), a multisystem disorder dominated by skeletal anomalies and (4) Alzheimer disease type 3. In this review we will discuss briefly the NOTCH subtypes and will concentrate on NOTCH3 in specific, taking in consideration its involvement in CADASIL syndrome.[70]

NOTCH1–associated with Congenital Heart Disease (CHD)

Garg et al. [71] first observed the involvement of the Notch1 receptor gene with CHD by studying two families with heterozygous mutations whose main feature was bicuspid aortic valve (BAV) and calcification.

Mutations in Notch1 in CHD in human are considered to be a susceptibility factor, rather than playing an essential role in terms of Mendelian disease. Urbanek et al.[72] have observed in a study conducted on cardiac stem cells (CSCs) in newborn mice, a presence of Nkx2.5 (a protein important to cardiac development, and mutations in the gene are associated with human CHD), coupled with the Notch1 intracellular domain in one multipotent cell line CSCs.[72] Furthermore, NOTCH1 has been associated with gastric cancer and was observed in both premalignant and malignant tissues.[73] Moreover, Notch1 may play a vital role in both encouraging metaplastic transition of gastric epithelial cells and in the preservation of proliferating intestinalised epithelial cells.[73]

NOTCH2 - Multisystem Disorder (Skeletal Effects)

Mutations in Notch2 pathway genes are associated with two multisystem disorders, namely ALGS (Alagille syndrome) and HJCYS (Hajdu–Cheney syndrome). Roughly 1% of ALGS is caused by mutated NOTCH2, which is also the only known gene linked to HJCYS.[74]

The finding of NOTCH2 mutations was a breakthrough for exome sequencing in two different studies conducted by Simpson and Isidor. [75,76] All reported mutations occur in exon 34, which is the last exon of NOTCH2, and all are predicted to lead to shortening of the protein product.[75,76]

NOTCH3 – CADASIL

NOTCH3 (N3) is a member of the Notch receptor family, which regulates cell destiny during embryonic development[77] and is chiefly present in vascular smooth muscle cells (VSMC) in adulthood.[8, 78] The human *NOTCH3* gene consists of 33 exons extending roughly 7 kb, was mapped to chromosome 19q13.1–13.26, and encodes a transmembrane protein comprising 2321 amino acids.[79]

NOTCH3 is a membrane-spanning protein with a large extracellular domain (N3ECD) containing 34 epidermal growth factor-like (EGF-like) repeats and a smaller intracellular domain with six ankyrin repeats. Each EGF-like domain contains six conserved cysteine residues, [18] which are vital for the correct folding of the EGF-like repeats and possibly for the function of the receptor.[80] An increasing body of evidence suggests that ligand-induced Notch signalling plays a pivotal role, both in various developmental contexts during embryonic development and also in adult tissues.[80] However, the specific role of Notch3 signalling in different developmental paradigms remains unclear and its function is not crucial for embryonic development but is needed after birth. NOTCH3 directs postnatal arterial maturation and helps to maintain arterial integrity. It is involved in regulation of vascular tone and in the wound healing of a vascular injury. In addition, NOTCH3 promotes cell survival by inducing expression of anti-apoptotic proteins.

In 1996, Joute et al identified a human gene mutation in NOTCH3 as the malfunctioning gene causing CADASIL pathology.[8, 81]

The majority of mutations in the NOTCH3 gene in patients with CADASIL are located in exon 4, followed by exons 3, 5, 6 and 11, and mutations are present in 50% of cases. All CADASIL-causing mutations identified so far are located in the EGF-like domains of *NOTCH3* and the majority of the mutations cause gain or loss of one cysteine residue in one of these repeats leading to an odd number of cysteine residues, which in turn leads to misfolding of N3ECD. This misfolding most likely alters the maturation, targetting, degradation and/or function of the NOTCH3 receptor.[80, 82, 83]

NOTCH4 - Metastatic Melanoma

Notch4 may play a crucial role in the equilibrium of cell growth and regulation of the aggressive phenotype and functions of Nodal which has been demonstrated in the study of Hardy et al.,[84] as a regulator of aggressive tumor cells in metastatic Melanoma, for studies have showed a very close correlation between Notch4 and Nodal expression in multiple aggressive cell lines.[84]

Conclusions

Germline mutations in Notch pathway genes give rise to a array of syndromes which, presently, can be clustered into: (1) The spondylocostal dysostosis (SCD); (2) Alagille syndrome (ALGS), NOTCH1-related congenital heart disease (CHD) and CADASIL; (3) Hajdu–Cheney syndrome (HJCYS), a multisystem disorder dominated by skeletal anomalies and (4) Alzheimer disease type 3. In this review we will discuss briefly the NOTCH subtypes and will concentrate on NOTCH3 in specific, taking in consideration its involvement in CADASIL syndrome, [70] development and is chiefly present in vascular smooth muscle cells (VSMC) in adulthood. Mutations in NOTCH3 create the malfunctioning gene causing CADASIL pathology.

CADASIL is the most common form of hereditary subcortical vascular dementia. The main clinical features are migraine with aura (often atypical or isolated), strokes, cognitive decline, dementia, and psychiatric symptoms. Smooth muscle cells in the small arteries throughout the body degenerate and vessel walls become fibrotic. In the brain, this results in circulatory disturbances and lacunar infarcts, mainly in the cerebral white matter and deep gray matter.

References

1. Tikka S, Mykkanen K, Ruchoux MM, Bergholm R, Junna M, Poyhonen M: Congruence between NOTCH3 mutations and GOM in 131 CADASIL patients. *Brain* 2009; **132**:933–939.

2. Arboleda-Velasquez JF, Lopera F, Lopez E: C455R NOTCH3 mutation in a Colombian CADASIL kindred with early onset of stroke. *Neurology* 2002; **59**:277–279.

3. Opherk C, Peters N, Herzog J, Luedtke R, Dichgans M: Long-term prognosis and causes of death in CADASIL: a retrospective study in 411 patients. *Brain* 2004;**127**:2533–2539.

4. Singhal S, Bevan S, Barrick T: The influence of genetic and cardiovascular risk factors on the CADASIL phenotype. *Brain* 2004;**127**:2031–2038.

5. Federico A, Bianchi S, Dotti MT: The spectrum of mutations for CADASIL diagnosis. *Neurol Sci* 2005; **26**:117–124.

6. Sourander P, Walinder J: Hereditary multi-infarct dementia. Morphological and clinical studies of a new disease. *Acta Neuropathol 1977;* **39**:247-54.

7. Tournier-Lasserve E, Joutel A, Melki J, Weissenbach J, Lathrop GM, Chabriat H, et al. Cerebral autosomal dominant arteriopathy with subcortical infarcts and leukoencephalopathy maps to chromosome 19q12. *Nat Genet.* 1993;3(3):256-9.

8. Joutel A, Corpechot C, Ducros A: *Notch3* mutations in CADASIL, a hereditary late-onset condition causing stroke and dementia. *Nature* 1996; **383**: 707-710.

9. Tikka S, Peng Ng, Di Maio G, Mykkänen K, Siitonen M, Lepikhova T: CADASIL mutations and shRNA silencing of NOTCH3 affect actin organization in cultured vascular smooth muscle cells. *Journal of Cerebral Blood Flow & Metabolism* 2012; **32**: 2171-2180.

10. Kalimo H, Miao Q, Tikka S, Mykkanen K, Junna M, Roine S: CADASIL: the most common hereditary subcortical vascular dementia. *Future Neurol* 2008; **3**: 683–704.

11. Ayata C: CADASIL: experimental insights from animal models. Stroke 2010; **41**(10 Suppl): S129-34. doi: 10.1161/STROKEAHA.110.595207.

12. Shahien R, Bianchi S, and Bowirrat A: Cerebral autosomal dominant arteriopathy with subcortical infarcts and leukoencephalopathy (CADASIL); Familiar study and review of the literature. *Neuropsychiatric disease and treatment* 2011; **7**: 383–390.

13. Dong Y, Hassan A, Zhang Z, Huber D, Dalageorgou C, Markus HS: Yield of screening for CADASIL mutations in lacunar stroke and leukoaraiosis. *Stroke* 2003; **34**:203–205.

14. Chabriat H, Vahedi K, Iba-Zizen MT, Joutel A, Nibbio A, Nagy TG: Clinical spectrum of CADASIL: a study of 7 families. Cerebral autosomal dominant arteriopathy with subcortical infarcts and leukoencephalopathy. *Lancet* 1995; **346**:934–939.

15. Tournier-Lasserve E, Joutel A, Melki J: Cerebral autosomal dominant arteriopathy with subcortical infarcts and leukoencephalopathy maps to chromosome 19q12. *Nat Genet* 1993; **3**:256–259.

16. Sourander P, Walinder J: Hereditary multi-infarct dementia. Morphological and clinical studies of a new disease. *Acta Neuropathol* 1977; **39**:247–254.

17. Stevens DL, Hewlett RH, Brownell B: Chronic familial vascular encephalopathy. *Lancet* 1977;**1**: 364–365.

18. Chabriat H, Vahedi K, Iba-Zizen MT: Clinical spectrum of CADASIL: a study of 7 families. Cerebral autosomal dominant arteriopathy with subcortical infarcts and leukoencephalopathy. *Lancet* 1995; **346:** 934-939.

19. Dichgans M, Mayer M, Uttner I: The phenotypic spectrum of CADASIL: Clinical findings in 102 cases. *Ann. Neurol 1998;* **44**: 731-739.

20. Kalimo H and Kalaria RN: Hereditary forms of vascular dementias. In: *Pathology and Genetics: Cerebrovascular Diseases* . Kalimo H (Ed). *ISN Neuropath Press, Basel* 2005; **41**: 324-334.

21. Mykkänen K, Junna M, Amberla K: Different clinical phenotypes in monozygotic CADASIL twins with a novel NOTCH3 mutation. *Stroke* 2009; **40**:2215–2218.

22. Lee SJ, Meng H, Elmadhoun O, Blaivas M, Wang MM: Cerebral autosomal dominant arteriopathy with subcortical infarcts and leukoencephalopathy affecting an African American man: identification of a novel 15-base pair NOTCH3 duplication. *Arch Neurol* 2011; **68**: 1584-1586. doi: 10.1001/archneurol.2011.781.

23. Dichgans M: "Quantitative MRI in CADASIL Correlation with disability and cognitive performance." *Neurology* 1999; **52**: 1361-1361.

24. Chabriat H: "Patterns of MRI lesions in CADASIL." *Neurology* 1998; **51**: 452-457.

25. Dichgans M: CADASIL: a monogenic condition causing stroke and subcortical vascular dementia. *Cerebrovascular Disease* 2002; **13:** 37–41.

26. Pfefferkorn T, von Stuckrad-Barre S, Herzog J: Reduced cerebrovascular CO(2) reactivity in CADASIL: a transcranial Doppler sonography study. *Stroke* 2001; **32**: 17–21.

27. Menon S, Cox HC, Kuwahata M: Association of a Notch 3 gene polymorphism with migraine susceptibility. *Cephalalgia* 2011;**31**: 264–270.

28. Valenti R, Poggesi F, Pescini D, Inzitari LP: Psychiatric disturbances in CADASIL: a brief review. *Acta Neurol Scand* 2008;**118**:291–295.

29. Chabriat H, Joutel A, Dichgans M, Tournier-Lasserve E, Bousser M-G. CADASIL. *Lancet Neurol.* 2009; **8**: 643–653.

30. Soyeon Park, Boram Park, Min Kyung Koh and Ho Joo: Case report: bipolar disorder as the first manifestation of Cadasil. *BMC Psychiatry* 2014; **14**:175.

31. Adib-Samii P, Brice G,Martin RJ, Markus HS: Clinical spectrum of CADASIL and the effect of cardiovascular risk factors on phenotype: study in 200 consecutively recruited individuals. *Stroke* 2010; **41**: 630–634.

32. Dichgans M, Ludwig H, Muller-Hocker J, Messerschmidt A, Gasser T: Small in-frame deletions and missense mutations in CADASIL: 3D models predict misfolding of NOTCH3 EGF-like repeat domains. *Eur J Hum Genet* 2000; **8**: 280–285.

33. Dichgans M, Herzog J, Gasser T. NOTCH3 in-frame deletion involving three cysteine residues in a family with typical CADASIL. *Neurology* 2001;**57**:1714–1717.

34. Joutel A, Vahedi K, Corpechot C: Strong clustering and stereotyped nature of NOTCH3 mutations in CADASIL patients. *Lancet* 1997; **350**: 1511–1515.

35. Joutel A, Chabriat H, Vahedi K: Splice site mutation causing a seven amino acid NOTCH3 in-frame deletion in CADASIL. *Neurology* 2000; **54**:1874–1875.

36. Federico A, Bianchi S, Dotti MT. The spectrum of mutations for CADASIL diagnosis. *Neurol Sci* 2005; **26**:117–124.

37. Arboleda-Velasquez JF, Lopera F, Lopez E: C455R NOTCH3 mutation in a Colombian CADASIL kindred with early onset of stroke. *Neurology* 2002; **59**: 277–279.

38. Opherk C, Peters N, Herzog J, Luedtke R, Dichgans M: Long-term prognosis and causes of death in CADASIL: a retrospective study in 411 patients. *Brain* 2004;**127**:2533–2539.

39. Tuominen S, Juvonen V, Amberla K, et al. Phenotype of a homozygous CADASIL patient in comparison to 9 age matched heterozygous patients with the same R133C NOTCH3 mutation. *Stroke* 2001; **32**: 1767–1774.

40. Dotti MT, Bianchi S, De Stefano N: Screening for CADASIL mutations in leukoencephalopathies. *Neurology* 2003; **60**:A89.

41. Liem MK, Lesnik Oberstein SA, Vollebregt MJ: Homozygosity for a NOTCH3 mutation in a 65-year-old CADASIL patient with mild symptoms: a family report. *J Neurol* 2009; **255**:1978–1980.

42. Joutel A, Dodick DD, Parisi JE, Cecillon M, Tournier-Lasserve E, Bousser MG: De novo mutation in the NOTCH3 gene causing CADASIL. *Ann Neurol* 2000; **47**:388–391.

43. Coto E, Menendez M, Navarro R, Garcia-Castro M, Alvarez V: A new de novo NOTCH3 mutation causing CADASIL. *Eur J Neurol* 2006;**13**: 628–631.

44. Kim Y, Cho EJ, Cho CG. Characteristics of CADASIL in Korea: a novel cysteine-sparing Notch3 mutation. *Neurology* 2006; **66**: 1511–1516.

45. Karlstrom H, Beatus P, Dannaeus K, Chapman G, Lendahl U, Lundkvist J: A CADASIL mutated NOTCH3 receptor exhibits impaired intracellular trafficking and maturation but normal ligand-induced signaling. *Proc Natl Acad Sci* 2002; **99**:17119–17124.

46. Davous P: CADASIL: a review with proposed diagnostic criteria. *Eur J Neurol* 1998; **5**:219–233.

47. Bogaert V: Rapidly evolving progressive subcortical encephalopathy of Binswanger's type in two sisters. *Med Hellen* 1955; **24**:961–972.

48. Bousser MG, Tournier-Lasserve E. Summary of the proceedings of the First International Workshop on CADASIL. *Stroke* 1994; **25**: 704–707.

49. Low WC, Junna M, Borjesson-Hanson A: Hereditary multiinfarct dementia of the Swedish type is a novel disorder different from NOTCH3 causing CADASIL. *Brain* 2007; **130**:357–367.

50. Sonninen V, Savontaus ML: Hereditary multi-infarct dementia. *Eur Neurol* 1987; **27**:209–215.

51. Opherk C, Peters N, Herzog J, Luedtke R, Dichgans M: Long-term prognosis and causes of death in CADASIL: a retrospective study in 411 patients. *Brain* 2004;**127**:2533–2539.

52. Kalimo H, Miao Q, Tikka S, et al. CAASIL: the most common hereditary subcortical vascular dementia. *Future Neurol* 2008; **3**:683–704.

53. Mykkanen K, Savontaus ML, Juvonen V: Detection of the founder effect in Finnish CADASIL families. *Eur J Hum Genet* 2004; **12**: 813–819.

54. Markus HS, Martin RJ, Simpson MA: Diagnostic strategies in CADASIL. *Neurology* 2002; **59**:1134–1138.

55. Oberstein SA. Diagnostic strategies in CADASIL. *Neurology*. 2003;60: 2020.

56. Oberstein SA. Diagnostic strategies in CADASIL. *Neurology* 2003; **60**: 2020.

57. Peters N, Opherk C, Bergmann T, Castro M, Herzog J, Dichgans M: Spectrum of mutations in biopsy-proven CADASIL: implications for diagnostic strategies. *Arch Neurol* 2005; **62**:1091–1094.

58. Arboleda-Velasquez JF, Lopera F, Lopez E: C455R NOTCH3 mutation in a Colombian CADASIL kindred with early onset of stroke. *Neurology* 2002; **59**:277–279.

59. van den Boom R, Lesnik Oberstein SA, Ferrari MD, Haan J, van Buchem MA: Cerebral autosomal dominant arteriopathy with subcortical infarcts and leukoencephalopathy: MR imaging findings at different ages – 3rd–6th decades. *Radiology* 2003; **229**:683–690.

60. Singhal S, Bevan S, Barrick T, Rich P, Markus HS: The influence of genetic and cardiovascular risk factors on the CADASIL phenotype. *Brain* 2004;**127**:2031–2038.

61. Dotti MT, Federico A, Mazzei R, et al. The spectrum of NOTCH3 mutations in 28 Italian CADASIL families. *J Neurol Neurosurg Psychiatry* 2005;**76**:736–738.

62. Pradotto L, Azan G, Doriguzzi C, Valentini C, Mauro A: Sporadic vascular dementia as clinical presentation of a new missense mutation within exon 7 of NOTCH3 gene. *J Neurol Sci* 2008; **271**:207–210.

63. Stromillo ML, Dotti MT, Battaglini M. Structural and metabolic brain abnormalities in preclinical cerebral autosomal dominant arteriopathy with subcortical infarcts and leucoencephalopathy. *J Neurol Neurosurg Psychiatry* 2009; **80**:41–47.

64. Bohlega S, Al Shubili A, Edris A: CADASIL in Arabs: clinical and genetic findings. *BMC Med Genet* 2007;**8**:67.

65. Ladi E, Nichols JT, Ge W: The divergent DSL ligand Dll3 does not activate NOTCH signaling but cell autonomously attenuates signaling induced by other DSL ligands. *J Cell Biol* 2005;**170**:983–992.

66. Fleming RJ: Structural conservation of NOTCH receptors and ligands. *Semin Cell Dev Biol* 1998; **9**:599–607.

67. Yoon K, Gaiano N: NOTCH signaling in the mammalian central nervous system: insights from mouse mutants. *Nat Neurosci* 2005; **8**:1411.

68. Shawber CJ, Kitajewski J: NOTCH function in the vasculature: insights from zebrafish, mouse and man. *Bioessays* 2004; **26**:225–234.

69. Morgan TH: The theory of the Gene. *American Naturalist* 1917; **51**: 513–544.

70. Turnpenny PD: Syndromes and Diseases Associated with the Notch Signalling Pathway. In: eLS. John Wiley & Sons, Ltd: 2014 Chichester.

71. Garg V, Muth AN, Ransom JF: Mutations in NOTCH1 cause aortic valve disease. *Nature* 2005; **437**: 270–274.

72. Urbanek K, Cabral-da-Silva MC, Ide-Iwata N: Inhibition of notch1-dependent cardiomyogenesis leads to a dilated myopathy in the neonatal heart. *Circulation Research* 2010; **107**: 429–441.

73. Brzozowa M, Mielanczyk L, Michalski M: Role of Notch signaling pathway in gastric cancer pathogenesis. *Contemporary Oncology (Poznan', Poland)* 2013; **17**: 1–5.

74. Sun Y, Gao X, Liu J: Differential Notch1 and Notch2 expression and frequent activation of Notch signaling in gastric cancers. *Archives of Pathology & Laboratory Medicine* 2011; **135**: 451–458.

75. Simpson MA, Irving MD, Asilmaz E: Mutations in NOTCH2 cause Hajdu-Cheney syndrome, a disorder of severe and progressive bone loss. Nature Genetics 2011; **43**: 303–305.

76. Isidor B, Lindenbaum P, Pichon O: Truncating mutations in the last exon of NOTCH2 cause a rare skeletal disorder with osteoporosis. *Nature Genetics* 2011; **43**: 306–308.

77. Artavanis-Tsakonas S, Rand MD, Lake RJ: Notch signaling: cell fate control and signal integration in development. *Science* 1999: **284**: 770–776.

78. Joutel A, Andreux F, Gaulis S, Domenga V, Cecillon M: The ectodomain of the Notch3 receptor accumulates within the cerebrovasculature of CADASIL patients. *J Clin Invest* 2000: **105**: 597–605.

79. Ungaro C, Mazzei R, Conforti FL: Cadasil: extended polymorphisms and mutational analysis of the NOTCH3 gene. *J Neurosci Res* 2009; **87**:1162–1167.

80. Artavanis-Tsakonas S, Matsuno K, Fortini M: Notch signalling. *Science* 1995; **268**: 225–232.

81. Larsson C, Lardelli M, White I, Lendahl U: The human NOTCH1, 2, and 3 genes are located at chromosome positions 9q34, 1p13-p11, and 19p13.2-p13.1 in regions of neoplasia-associated translocation. *Genomics* 1994; **24**:253–258.

82. Desmond DW, Moroney JT, Lynch T *et al*: CADASIL in a North American family; clinical, pathologic and radiologic findings. *Neurology* 1998; **51**: 844– 849.

83. Mellies JK, Bäumer T, Müller JA: SPECT study of a German CADASIL family: a phenotype with migraine and progressive dementia only. *Neurology* 1998; **50**: 1715–1721.

84. Hardy KM, Kirschmann DA, Seftor EA: Regulation of the embryonic morphogen Nodal by Notch4 facilitates manifestation of the aggressive melanoma phenotype. *Cancer Research* 2010; **70**:10340–10350.

Figure 1: The exonic structure of the human NOTCH3 gene and the domains of the NOTCH3 receptor protein.

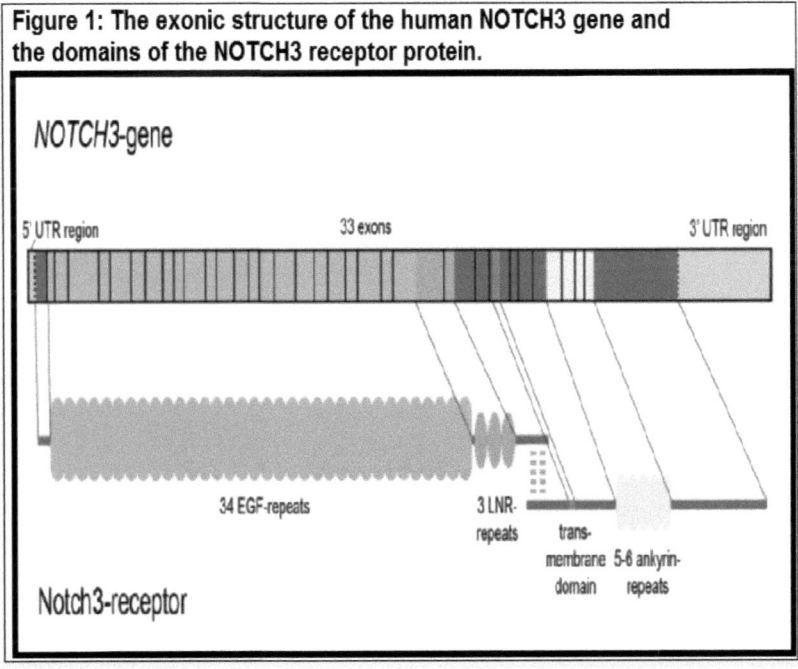

Figure 2: The symptom manifestation and findings in CADASIL during the disease course. WM; White Matter, MRI; Magnetic Resonance Imaging, GOM; Granular Osmiophilic Material.

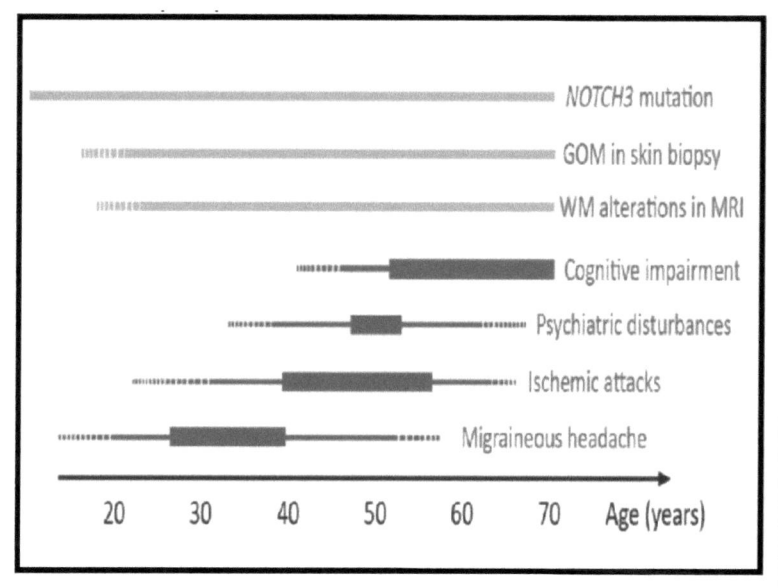

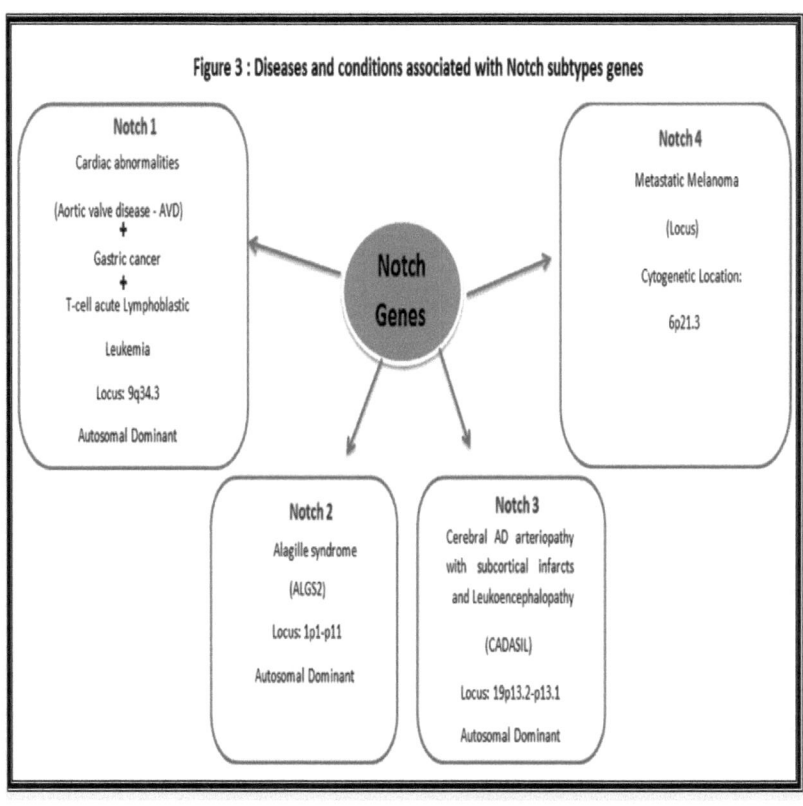

Figure 3 : Diseases and conditions associated with Notch subtypes genes

Notch 1

Cardiac abnormalities

(Aortic valve disease - AVD)
+
Gastric cancer
+
T-cell acute Lymphoblastic

Leukemia

Locus: 9q34.3

Autosomal Dominant

Notch Genes

Notch 4

Metastatic Melanoma

(Locus)

Cytogenetic Location:

6p21.3

Notch 2

Alagille syndrome

(ALGS2)

Locus: 1p1-p11

Autosomal Dominant

Notch 3

Cerebral AD arteriopathy with subcortical infarcts and Leukoencephalopathy

(CADASIL)

Locus: 19p13.2-p13.1

Autosomal Dominant

CHAPTER 2 - The Pathogenesis of CADASIL.

Introduction

CADASIL is essentially a microangiopathy disorder affecting essentially the brain and is the most common monogenic form of hereditary cerebral microangiopathy disorder manifesting usually in early adulthood. To date, more than 200 mutations of *NOTCH* homolog *3* gene, located on chromosome-19p13.1–13.26., have been reported in CADASIL patients.[1-3] Over 95% of the mutations are mapped in EGF-like repeat domain of NOTCH3 [data from HGMD]. Almost all of the mutations are missense and lead to either gain or loss of a Cysteine residue, causing an odd number of Cysteine and further misfolding of the EGF-like repeat domain. This misfolding may change the maturation, targeting, degradation and function of the NOTCH3 receptor, which plays a key role for most phenotypes of CADASIL affected families.

CADASIL is a dominantly inherited neurodegenerative disease and the most common cause of hereditary pure vascular dementia. Penetrance of the disease is probably 100%, but expression varies in age of onset, severity of the clinical symptoms, and progression of the disease. Affected individuals exhibit a variety of symptoms, and clinical presentation of CADASIL varies even among and within families. The main symptoms are an early recurrent ischemic strokes (84%), subcortical vascular dementia (80%), migraine with atypical aura (35%), and psychiatric disturbances (20%). The pathological hallmarks of CADASIL are profound demyelination and axonal damage, as well as arteriopathy involving distinctive degeneration of the arterial smooth muscle cells in the brain and peripheral organs.[4] Gradual destruction of vascular smooth muscle cells (VSMCs) leads to progressive wall thickening, fibrosis, luminal narrowing in small and medium-sized penetrating arteries. The reduced cerebral blood flow finally causes lacunar infarcts, mainly in the basal ganglia and fronto-temporal white matter, which leads to cognitive impairments and dementia. Additionally, other hallmarks of the disease are the widespread vasculopathy, and the pathognomonic accumulation within the tunica media of arterial walls of granular osmiophilic material (GOM)[5] which is distinct from arteriosclerotic and amyloid angiopathy generally affecting leptomeningeal. Skin biopsy typically shows ultrastructural alterations of skin vessels similar to those of brain arteries.[6-8] Imaging abnormalities in CADASIL develop as the disease progresses.[9]

Magnetic Resonance Imaging (MRI) hyperintensities signals in subcortical white matter and basal ganglia, are consistently visualized from age 21 years onward.[10] In patients aged 20-30 years with a pathogenic mutation, typical white matter hyperintensities first appear in the anterior temporal lobes, but the rest of the white matter, except for periventricular caps, appear unaffected.[10] Affected patients' white matter hyperintensities are symmetrically distributed and located in the periventricular and deep white matter.

Within the white matter, the frontal lobe is the site with the highest lesion load, followed by the temporal and parietal lobes[11] and Subcortical lacunar lesions (SLLs). Linearly arranged groups of rounded, circumscribed lesions at the junction of the grey and white matter with signal intensity identical to that of cerebrospinal fluid and SLLs are found in approximately two-thirds of affected patients and may be a specific marker for CADASIL.[12] Cerebral microbleeds are located predominantly in the thalamus and are best visualized with T2 - weighted gradient echo imaging.[13]

NOTCH3 gene mutation causes CADASIL Pathology

Mutations in NOTCH3 have been identified as the underlying cause of CADASIL. NOTCH3 gene is located in the short arm of chromosome 19q13.1–13.26,[14] and it is a large (~41.3 kilobase) gene containing 33 exons. The gene is 2321 amino acids glycosylated transmembrane receptor.[14] The identification of a pathogenic NOTCH3 mutation is an indisputable evidence for CADASIL, until today, it is known over 200 different NOTCH3 gene defects.[1-3, 15]

Pathogenic mutations in CADASIL patients identified to date are predominantly missense mutations within the NOTCH3 extracellular domain, which either add or delete Cysteine residues resulting in an odd number of Cysteines.[16] This is believed to promote abnormal Cysteine-Cysteine interactions leading to conformational changes, pathological homo/heterodimerization or multimerization.[17-19] Indeed, in CADASIL, NOTCH3 extracellular domain accumulates in the cytoplasmic membrane of VSMCs.[17, 18-21] This gene encodes the third discovered human homologue of the Drosophilia melanogaster type I membrane protein notch. Four different Notch receptors (Notch 1—4) and five Notch ligands (Deltalike-1,-3,-4, Jagged-1,-2) have been identified in mammals. Notch signaling has an essential role in different developmental events during the embryonic development as well as in adult tissues. In mammals, Notch3 signaling influences cell-destiny decisions by regulating gene expression, cell differentiation, proliferation, and apoptosis and is periodically expressed in many different tissues in several phases of the embryonic development.

In addition, the regulation of neurogenesis, myogenesis, angiogenesis, haematopoiesis and epithelial–mesenchymal transition are all crucially influenced by Notch signaling. In the adult human, the *NOTCH3* gene is expressed almost exclusively in the VSMCs[22] and plays a crucial roles in postnatal differentiation, maturation and phenotypic behavior of VSMCs, regulation of VSMCs growth and apoptosis, response to vascular injury, and regulation of actins cytoskeleton in response to mechanical stretching of the vessel wall by intraluminal pressure.[23-25]

Conclusions

The Notch signaling pathway indicates a very complicated cell interaction mechanism, playing an essential part in metazoan development, which ultimately determines cell destinies in regards of differentiation, proliferation and apoptosis. CADASIL is a rare autosomal dominant disease that is essentially a micro-angiopathy affecting mainly the brain and is caused by mutations in NOTCH3 gene located in the short arm of chromosome 19. Most mutations in the NOTCH3 gene in patients with CADASIL are located in exon 4, followed by exons 3, 5, 6 and 11, and mutations are found in over 90% of cases.[26-28] Geographic variations have been described, showing variability in the distribution of the disease worldwide, for example, mutations in exon 3 of the NOTCH3 gene represent the second most common mutation site in the French, British and German populations, whereas mutations in exon 11 are more frequently seen in the Dutch.[26-28]

CADASIL is the most common cause of hereditary stroke, hereditary pure vascular dementia and disabling systemic condition in adulthood, characterized by migraine with aura, recurrent lacunar strokes, progressive cognitive impairment, and psychiatric disorders. The clinical presentation of CADASIL is heterogeneous, and may be confused with multiple sclerosis, Alzheimer dementia, and Binswanger disease, that's why an accurate differential diagnosis is needed. The specific clinical signs and symptoms, along with genetic testing and brain MRI findings, are essential in determining the diagnosis of CADASIL. When the differential diagnosis includes

CADASIL, various other tests are available for diagnosis such as: Immunohistochemistry assay of a skin biopsy sample, detection of granular osmiophilic material (GOM) in the same skin biopsy sample by electron microscopy. Genetic testing, by direct sequencing of selected exons or of exons 2-24 of the NOTCH3 gene is also important for the diagnosis.

References

1. Shahien R, Bianchi S, and Bowirrat A: Cerebral autosomal dominant arteriopathy with subcortical infarcts and leukoencephalopathy (CADASIL); Familiar study and review of the literature. *Neuropsychiatric disease and treatment* 2011; 7: 383–390.

2. Joutel A. Pathogenesis of CADASIL: transgenic and knockout mice to probe function and dysfunction of the mutated gene, Notch3, in the cerebrovasculature. *Bioessays* 2010;33:73-80.

3. Ge W, Kuang H, Wei B, Bo L, Xu Z, et al. A Novel Cysteine-Sparing *NOTCH3* Mutation in a Chinese Family with CADASIL. *PLoS ONE* 2014; 9: e104533. doi:10.1371/journal.pone.0104533.

4. Adib-Samii P, Brice G, Martin RJ, Markus HS. Clinical spectrum of CADASIL and the effect of cardiovascular risk factors on phenotype: study in 200 consecutively recruited individuals. *Stroke* 2010;41:630-4.

5. Goebel HH, Meyermann R, Rosin R, Schlote W. Characteristic morphologic manifestation of CADASIL, cerebral autosomal- dominant arteriopathy with subcortical infarcts and leukoencephalopathy, in skeletal muscle and skin. Muscle Nerve 1997;20:625–7.

6. LaPoint SF, Patel U, Rubio A. Cerebral autosomal dominant arteriopathy with subcortical infarcts and leukoencephalopathy (CADASIL). *Adv Anat Pathol* 2000;7(5):307-21.

7. Malandrini A, Gaudiano C, Gambelli S, et al. Diagnostic value of ultrastructural skin biopsy studies in CADASIL. *Neurology* 2007;68(17):1430-1432.

8. Gutierrez-Molina M, Rodriguez AC, Garci CM, et al. Small arterial granular degeneration in familial Binswanger's syndrome. *Acta Neuropathol* 1994;87:98-105.

9. Liem MK, Lesnik Oberstein SA, Vollebregt MJ, Middelkoop HA, van der Grond J, Helderman-van den Enden AT. Homozygosity for a NOTCH3 mutation in a 65-year-old CADASIL patient with mild symptoms: a family report. J Neurol 2008b;255:1978–80.

10. Oberstein SAJ. Diagnostic strategies in CADASIL. Neurology 2003;60:2020.

11. O'Sullivan M, Jarosz JM, Martin RJ, et al. MRI hyperintensities of the temporal lobe and external capsule in patients with CADASIL. Neurology 2001;56:628–34.

12. van den Boom R, Lesnik Oberstein SA, van Duinen SG, et al. Subcortical lacunar lesions: an MR imaging finding in patients with cerebral autosomal dominant arteriopathy with subcortical infarcts and leukoencephalopathy. Radiology 2002;224:791–6.

13. Dichgans M, Holtmannspotter M, Herzog J, et al. Cerebral microbleeds in CADASIL: a gradient-echo magnetic resonance imaging and autopsy study. Stroke 2002;33:67–71.

14. Joutel A, Corpechot C, Ducros A: *Notch3* mutations in CADASIL, a hereditary late-onset condition causing stroke and dementia. *Nature* 1996; 383: 707-710.

15. Tikka S, Mykkanen K, Ruchoux MM, et al. Congruence between NOTCH3 mutations and GOM in 131 CADASIL patients. *Brain* 2009;132:933–939.

16. Peters N, Opherk C, Bergmann T, et al. Spectrum of mutations in biopsy-proven CADASIL: implications for diagnostic strategies. *Arch Neurol* 2005; 62: 1091–1094.

17. Dichgans M, Ludwig H, Muller-Hocker J, et al. Small in-frame deletions and missense mutations in CADASIL: 3D models predict misfolding of Notch3 EGF-like repeat domains. *Eur J Hum Genet 2000*; *8: 280*–285.

18. Donahue CP, Kosik KS. Distribution pattern of Notch3 mutations suggests a gain-of-function mechanism for CADASIL. *Genomics 2004*; *83*: 59–65.

19. Opherk C, Duering M, Peters N, Karpinska A, Rosner S, Schneider E, Bader B, Giese A, Dichgans M. CADASIL mutations enhance spontaneous multimerization of Notch3. Hum Mol Genet 2009; 18: 2761–2767.

20. Dichgans M, Ludwig H, Muller-Hocker J, Messerschmidt A, Gasser T. Small in-frame deletions and missense mutations in CADASIL: 3D models predict misfolding of Notch3 EGF-like repeat domains. Eur J Hum Genet 2000; 8: 280–285.

21. Donahue CP, Kosik KS. Distribution pattern of Notch3 mutations suggests a gain-of-function mechanism for CADASIL. Genomics 2004; 83: 59–65.

22. Joutel A, Andreux F, Gaulis S, et al. The ectodomain of the Notch3 receptor accumulates within the cerebrovasculature of CADASIL patients. *J Clin Invest* 2000a;105:597-605.

23. Domenga V, Fardoux P, Lacombe P, et al. *Notch3* is required for arterial identity and maturation of vascular smooth muscle cells. *Genes Dev* 2004; 18(22): 2730–2735.

24. Wang T, Baron M, Trump D. An overview of Notch3 function in vascular smooth muscle cells. *Prog Biophys Mol Biol* 2008;96:499–509.

26. Markus HS, Martin RJ, Simpson MA, et al. Diagnostic strategies in CADASIL. *Neurology*. 2002;59:1134-1138.

27. Joutel A, Vahedi K, Corpechot C, et al. Strong clustering and stereotyped nature of *Notch3* mutations in CADASIL patients. *Lancet*. 1997;350:1511-1515.

28. Razvi SS, Davidson R, Bone I, Muir KW. Diagnostic strategies in CADASIL [comment; letter]. *Neurology*. 2003;60:2019-2020.

CHAPTER 3 - Candidate Biomarkers and CSF Profiles for Alzheimer's disease and CADASIL.

Introduction

Alzheimer's disease (AD) is an insidious neurological disease and a genetically heterogeneous disorder causing dementia in elderly and leading to a massive burden on AD individuals, their families, and on social and health care systems [1].

Its diagnosis is subjective, confirmed AD diagnosed can be done only after brain samples are examined by either biopsy or autopsy, and it covers 50-60% of all dementia cases. It is predicted that, by 2050, the number of elderly individuals over the age 80 years will advance 370 million globally and that more than half of those aged 85 years or older will be diagnosed with AD [2].

The etiologies of AD are Multifactorial; where genetics and environmental risk factors work in concert to cause the disease [3, 4]. Neuropathological features of AD depends on finding extracellular accumulations of β-amyloid peptides (Aβ) that guide to neurotic plaque formation and intracellular neurofibrillary tangles of hyperphosphorylated tau (p-tau), and total tau protein (t-tau) [5].

Which all together represent well accepted biomarkers of AD [6, 7, 8]. However, there are plethoras of evidences that support the involvement of cerebrovascular dysfunction in AD in addition to its primary role in vascular causes of cognitive deficits observed in vascular dementia [9].

Importantly, the manifestation of the ischemic episodes and neurodegenerative pathology was demonstrated to have a great influence on the appearance of dementia, signifying mutual connections between ischemic event and neurodegeneration [10, 11].

Indeed, a new term, entitled vascular dementia (VaD), encompasses a less defined group of dementia patients having a mixture of vascular illnesses that mainly appear in adulthood and necessitate suitable methods for diagnosis and differential diagnosis [12].

The differential diagnosis between AD (the first common and perhaps best known cause of Dementia) and VaD (The commonest cause of dementia after Alzheimer's dementia) are still roughly problematic in clinical practice, despite the widely used diagnostic criteria to differentiate between the two disorders [13].

It is well known, that ischemic stroke which leads to interruption or harshly reduced of blood supply to part of the brain causes vascular cognitive impairments (VaD), also owing to cerebrovascular deficit dementia of Alzheimer's type will appears [14, 15, 16, 17].

Cognitively patients, with AD, show sometimes mixed degrees of associated vascular lesions in 30-60% of AD cases. In opposition, cognitively patients, with VaD, may carry 40%-70% of AD pathology, consequently impeding diagnosis precision [15, 16, 17]. Therefore, to eliminate this bewilderment and discrepancies in the diagnosis between the AD and VaD, it is worthy to shed light firstly on a disease that is a microangiopathy and represents VaD with clear milestones and features as is the case of Cerebral Autosomal Dominant Arteriopathy with Subcortical Infarcts and Leukoencephalopathy (CADASIL) [21].

Studying CADASIL CSF biomarkers profile, will help in the differential diagnosis between both diseases sharing the coexisting neurodegeneration, furthermore, CADASIL is a dominantly inherited mid-adult life neurodegenerative disease, which belongs to vasculopathies and symbolizes a genuine prototype of VaD that provides a valuable opportunity for studying its CSF biomarkers. Secondly, examining and evaluating the CSF biomarkers of AD compared to that of CADASIL [22, 23, 24]. The pathogenesis similarities between CADASIL and early onset AD come from the fact that in both diseases genetic mutations occur in early adulthood [25, 26, 27]. CADASIL mutations in NOTCH3 gene generate Neurotoxic protein aggregates (Granular Osmiophilic Material-GOM) in the surrounding area of Vascular Smooth Muscle Cells (VSMCs) causing degeneration in addition to loss of VSMCs causing degeneration and loss of VSMCs in small arteries and arterioles of white matter regions of the brain [28, 29, 30]. The deposition and discrepancy of clearance of the neurotoxic GOM lead to neurodegenerative subcortical dementia, similar to those attributed to mutant forms of the Amyloid Precursor Proteins (APP) and presenilins genes which cause overproduction and accumulations of the toxic Aβ42 protein in the brain and collapse of Aβ42 clearance mechanisms which lead to neurodegenerative cortical dementia (AD). Despite the presumed pathological similarities, substantial differences between the two phenomena may exist especially in the CSF neurochemical phenotypes [31]. Our advance knowledge of the underlying biochemical and genetic mechanisms that cause these diseases has encouraged significantly our effort to develop biomarkers. The discovery of novel diagnostic methods based on CSF neurochemical phenotypes and neuroimaging biomarkers of neurodegenerative diseases specific pathology increase the capability to supply efficient procedures of natural history, biological activity and markers of surrogate endpoints. Biomarkers should be also judged according to their power to predict disease development, clinical diversity, and variations among the population in order to get a swift evaluation and therefore description for new cures [32]. According to these principals we viewed the literature that has searched CSF total tau (t-tau), β-amyloid protein 1-42, and phosphorylated tau (p-tau) as diagnostic tests for AD and, for a genuine prototype of VaD (CADASIL) that provide a unique opportunity for studying their CSF biomarkers.

Overview of Biomarkers Properties

Access to molecular and biochemical markers of neurodegenerative diseases would complement clinical approaches, and further the goals of early and accurate diagnosis. Hence, the importance of the biological markers studies which are quantitative measurements that provide information about: intrinsic biological processes, a disease circumstances and risk of developing an illness (antecedent biomarkers); assist in diagnosing disease (diagnostic biomarkers); response to treatment (prognostic biomarkers), providing much-needed insight into preclinical and clinical data, all of these are still valid procedures for early detection of diseases [33].

Detection the subject's susceptibility to the disease prior to appearance of prodromal signs, and detection of neural dysfunction before irreversible cellular damage, will be tremendously valuable for developing; prevention and intervention strategies and early treatments. From here stems the truthfulness and reliability of biomarker to distinguish between normal and interested disease [34].

In fact, biomarkers are set of factors used to measure anatomic, physiologic, biochemical, pharmacological, or molecular parameters associated with the presence and severity of particular disease states or processes in humans and animals [35, 36].

These characteristics are pragmatically calculated and carefully assessed as indicators of natural biologic or pathogenic mechanisms or pharmacological reactions to a curative intervention [35, 36, 37].

Nowadays, definition of biomarker panels comprehensively augments our understanding to quantify risk, assess prognosis, and determine response to therapy [38]. Years ago, biomarkers were mainly considered physiological markers such as blood pressure or heart rate [39].

In addition, biomarkers are gaining an important value and are used as a tool in different disciplines such as in field of oncology, immunology, cardiovascular diseases and metabolic diseases [40]. Photocopy for molecular biomarker, for instance, increased prostate specific antigen (PSA) which considered generally as a molecular biomarker for prostate malignancy or acute prostate inflammation [41].

Biomarkers are also used as molecular indicators in many epidemiologic studies mainly in exploring viruses such as (Human papilloma virus (HPV) or particular procarcinogen markers of tobacco exposure such as 4 - (methylnitrosamino)- 1- (3-pyridyl)-1-butanone (NNK) [42, 43]. Also, Genomic biomarkers have principal role in investigation diseases; such as Apolipoproteine Epsilon-4 allele (APOE-ε4) for AD, and HLA for looking for narcolepsy, CD19, Sialophorin, CD11 integrin cluster, and IL-4 receptor – for Crohn's disease. Other methods and assays are used like; Serum or Spinal fluid substance, Neuroimaging and Physiologic parameters [44, 45, 46, 47].

A. Overview of the CSF Biomarkers for AD and CADASIL.

CADASIL gene located at Chromosome 19p13.2.

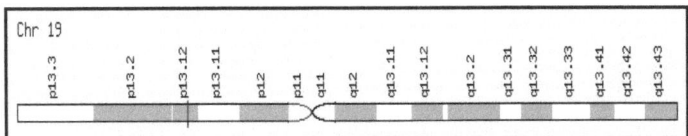

Plethora of biomarkers has been evaluated for AD. According to the literature more than 25 potential biomarkers for AD had previously been identified and new ones are still under investigation [48]. The CSF is a mirror of many processes that occur in the brain and its importance as a reasonable and direct target for many medical investigations (either physiological or pathological) comes from its straight communication with the brain, where many metabolic processes take place [49, 50].

In view of the fact, that AD pathology is chiefly limited to the brain, CSF is an apparent source and justified biomarkers for AD [51, 52].

Indeed, early biomarker discovery efforts for AD are based on concentration abnormalities of proteins such as β-amyloid 1-42, total tau protein, and phosphorylated tau (181,199,231) protein in CSF [53]. These CSF classical biomarkers reflect the neuropathological alterations occurring in AD brains, thus revealing the disease in its presymptomatic stage. However, it has been demonstrated that variations in the levels of these biomarkers in the CSF also appear in different degrees in other neurological diseases such as stroke, VaD and CADASIL. With the aim to investigate the utility of these biomarkers in the differential diagnosis between the various pathologies mentioned above and to evaluate the power of each biomarker and/or their combination in predicting different diseases progression, we have compared the levels of these CSF biomarkers in AD, VaD and CADASIL.

B. Amyloid βeta (Aβ)

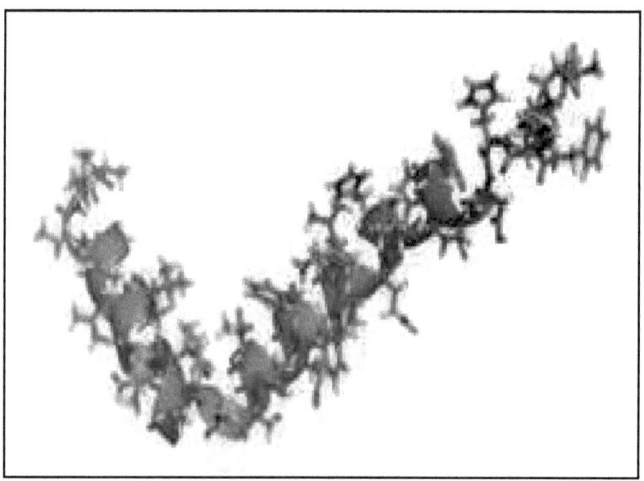

Although the production pathways and the absolute function of Aβ in the brain still vague, its presence as a main component of senile plaques is unambiguous. Aβ is created by a cluster of peptides formed by proteolytic cleavage of the type I transmembrane straddling glucoprotein amyloid precursor protein (APP, OMIM

104760, chromosome 21q21) through sequential cleavages by BACE1 (The major β-secretase in the brain) and γ-secretase complex [54, 55].

Missense mutations in the genes of APP and presenilins (*PSEN1*, OMIM 104311, chromosome 14q24.3) and presenilin 2 (*PSEN2*, OMIM 600759, chromosome 1q31-q42) genes that are located on chromosomes 21, 14, and 1, respectively exhibit the usual feature of altering the γ-secretase cleavage of APP to enhance the creation of the amyloidogenic Aβ42, the most important constituent of amyloid plaques in both genetic and sporadic AD [56, 57]. Paradoxically, "non-amyloidogenic pathway", APP is first sliced by the α-secretase, members of the ADAM (a disintegrin and metalloprotease) family of zinc metalloproteases, within the Aβ sequence thus precluding production of intact Aβ peptides [58].

The peptides, particularly Aβ1–42, are aggregation prone, self-assembling to form a heterogeneous mixture of soluble oligomers, protofibrils and fibrils. Only levels of the soluble, fibrillar oligomers were found to be elevated significantly in AD brains, where their levels correlate strongly with AD onset-severity, and are therefore proposed to be the major neurotoxic species in AD [59].

Consequent deleterious effects include neurotoxicity, memory impairments, inhibition of long-term potentiation (LTP), loss of dendritic spines and synaptic dysfunction [60].

Although the function of APP needs to be completely clarified, comprehending APP trafficking and processing may open new insights into the regulatory mechanism of the amyloidogenic pathway [61].

The processing of APP includes various stages, including APP sorting, transport, internalization and sequential proteolysis [62].

Distorted steering of APP trafficking and distribution in neurons might lead to the amyloidogenic pathway, which is implicated in the pathology of AD [63, 64].

Therefore, the intracellular distribution and transport of APP are crucial for Aβ production [65, 66].

Indeed, increased Aβ42 production throughout life and faulty clearance of Aβ mechanisms lead to accumulation of oligomerization of Aβ42 in limbic and association cortices, due to the altered in the many proteases in the brain that take part in Aβ degradation and clearance including cathepsins, gelatinases, endopeptidases, aminopeptidase, neprilysin, serine protease, and insulin-degrading enzyme [67, 68]. Aβ42 makes up less than 10% of total Aβ and it is the initial and major component of amyloid plaque deposits in AD [69].

The detection that Aβ42 peptide forms the essential component of AD plaques and that is secreted by cells led to examinations of Aβ42 in the CSF. Previous studies showed a decline in CSF-Aβ42 to about 40–50% in AD patients compared to control levels [70].

It is not clear why Aβ42 is reduced in AD patients, but it is thought that its decrease reflects trapping of Aβ42 in the amyloid plaques in the brain. Indeed, studies suggest that decreased CSF Aß42 correlates well with the levels of amyloid plaques in the AD brain as determined by amyloid imaging [71].

Consistent with the amyloid cascade hypothesis, the pathogenesis of AD states that Aβ accumulation in the brain begins in the early prodromal stage of AD, and it is a key factor that initiates the neurodegenerative process. Accumulation of Aβ in the brain of presymptomatic AD patients results consequently in decreasing the level of CSF Aß42. Therefore, CSF biomarkers (Aß42) are changed very early giving the opportunity to detect AD patients at risk or to be used as indicators of disease progression in persons with mild cognitive decline (MCD) [72]. More correctly, pathological abnormalities of AD manifest approximately a decade before any clinical symptoms appearance [73].

Considering the diagnostic sensitivity and specificity levels of Aβ42 in CSF – AD patients that ranged between 80% and 90%, may enhance its use as potential test in combinations with other tests [74, 75, 76].

More than two decade ago a new broader term called vascular dementia (VaD) appeared on the screen as new cognitive impairments pathology connected with cerebrovascular pathologies that do not fulfill AD criteria [77]. New criteria and diagnostic standards for this new disorder were recognized and have gained the attention of the clinical neuroscientists [24, 78, 79, 80].

Intensive studies in this topic indicate that cerebrovascular diseases and AD share the same risk factors [81] and this notion enhanced the thought that simultaneous ischemic events and neurodegenerative pathology have a deep effect on the manifestation of dementia, signifying a strong relation between ischemia and neurodegeneration and point out that cerebrovascular risk factors are highly involved in the pathogenesis of AD [82, 83, 84, 85].

Indeed, Aβ has a strong impact on the occurrence of cerebrovascular dysfunction, which in turn influences cerebral amyloidogenesis [86]. In addition, the hypoxia-ischemia process caused by Aβ could decrease the blood perfusion; diminish vascular reserves, and increase the tendency to ischemic damage [87].

42

Additionally, hypo-perfusion and/or ischemia encourage the cutting of Aβ from the amyloid precursor protein (APP) by up-regulating β-secretase expression and action [88, 89, 90].

On the light of these findings we can conclude that ischemia events exacerbates Aβ accumulation in the brain by decreasing the major elimination pathway of this neurotoxic peptide and in the end its brain clearance [91, 92].

Plethora of facts that cerebrovascular dysfunction acts not only in VaD but also in AD, comes from the fact that both impair the neurovascular unit, boost the view that a remarkable overlapping is exist between VaD and AD not only in the underlying risk factors mentioned above, but may also in sharing some CSF neurochemical phenotypes abnormalities. For example, the CSF profile of Aβ proteins in patients with AD is highly decreased (A pathological decreased of amyloid β_{1-42} is considered at <450 pg/ml) but Aβ CSF levels in VaD have been reported to be reasonably decreased or significantly overlapping with AD [93].

Given that previous studies illustrated conflicting results in VaD,

we investigated CSF biomarkers in CADASIL, since CADASIL represents a model of pure subcortical vascular dementia occurring in early adulthood, and doubtfully to share associated onset age with that of AD and it is the most common single gene disorder leading to ischemic stroke, which specifically affects the cerebral small vessels causing hypo-perfusion, ischemia and inability of the cerebral vessels to auto-regulate [96], we can expect that CSF biomarkers, especially Aβ, t-tau and p-tau levels, sufficiently discriminate between AD on one hand and CADASIL on other hand.

C. Total tau (Microtubule-associated protein tau)

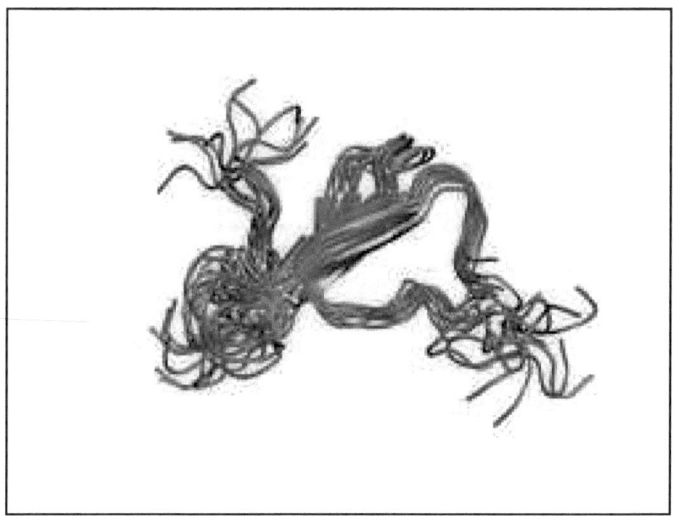

Even though the association of tau in the pathogenesis of neurodegenerative diseases has long been known, its specific mechanism of action in causing neural damage is still to be clarified [97].

Physiologically, tau proteins are an intracelluar microtubule-associated protein acting as stabilizers microtubules in the cell cytoskeleton, and pathologically, tau proteins characterize the main component relating to intraneuronal changes in AD patients.

Numerous new studies have doubted the hypothesis that filamentous tau that have accumulated are the most destructive forms of tau, and that tau deficiency is strongly involved in the pathogenesis of tauopathies. Novel discoveries suggest that tau regulates neuronal stimuli and that it is necessary for Aβ and other neurotoxins to cause neuronal deficits, unusual network activity and cognitive impairment [98].

Tau-Protein is a microtubule-associated protein situated in the neuronal axons. As a result of splicing of Tau-mRNA, there are six isoforms ranging in size from 352 to 441 amino acids, with molecular weights of around 50–65 kDa [99].

In normal situations, tau is synchronized by phosphorylation. In atypical conditions, tau turn into hyperphosphorylated (phospho-tau) and accumulates as paired helical filaments that combined into masses inside the neurons as neurofibrillary tangles (NFT), which symbolize one of the hallmarks of AD [100].

The logic for considering tau as biomarker is the presence of abnormal intraneuronal aggregates of phospho-tau observed in many tauopathies, including AD, Tau aggregates can be examined in the Brain and peripheral fluids. Biochemical and Immunohistochemical properties of Tau cumulative in brain permit postmortem categorization and differential diagnosis of tauopathies [101].

In 1993 the first report on CSF total-T as a biomarker for AD was offered. In that manuscript, an enzyme-linked immunosorbent assay (ELISA) with a polyclonal reporter antibody was used [102].

Total tau concentrations especially phosphorylated tau (181,199,231) proteins can be measured in the CSF as Aß, and show a good correlation with the diagnosis of AD [103].

Previous studies have established 300% increase in the concentration of total-Tau in CSF Alzheimer's patients 70 years and older versus control subjects younger than 50 years [(>600 pg/mL vs <200 pg/mL), respectively] [104].

A strong association between age and total-tau in healthy individuals has been determined with a cut off value of > 500 pg/mL (> 70 years) versus 450 pg/mL (< 70 years) [105].

CSF total-tau levels in AD patients have a sensitivity of 90% and specificity of 81% compared to healthy Control [106], compared to other dementias, the sensitivity and specificity drops to 50%-60% [107].

Notwithstanding, the relative high sensitivity and specificity that CSF T-tau level plays as discriminator between AD patients and control, its presence in other neurological diseases for instance, VaD, progressive supranuclear palsy, corticobasal degeneration, CADASIL, and its notable high concentration in Spongiform Encephalopathies (3000 pg/mL), decreases at some level its validity as AD specific biomarker [108, 109].

However, the absence of specific novel biomarker for AD and related disorders require a combination of different candidate's biomarkers. The decreased CSF levels of Aβ42 in AD, VaD and CADASIL enhance the effort to find additional biomarkers that may be utilized to differentiate between them. For this reason, we investigated changes in CSF biomarker profiles in patients with AD, VaD and CADASIL. Especially the changes in total tau, which plays a fundamental role in indicating neuronal damage, thus observed altered in CSF of AD and VaD patients.

The CSF outline of total tau in AD sufferers is characterized by increased levels. Researches on CSF biomarker in VaD illustrated contradictory results: total-tau levels have been showed to be augmented, intact, and intermediate or significantly overlapping with AD, whereas, in CADASIL, total-tau levels were intact and considerably dissimilar in comparison to AD.

D. <u>Human Phosphorylated tau (P-tau: phosphorylated at Thr181)</u>

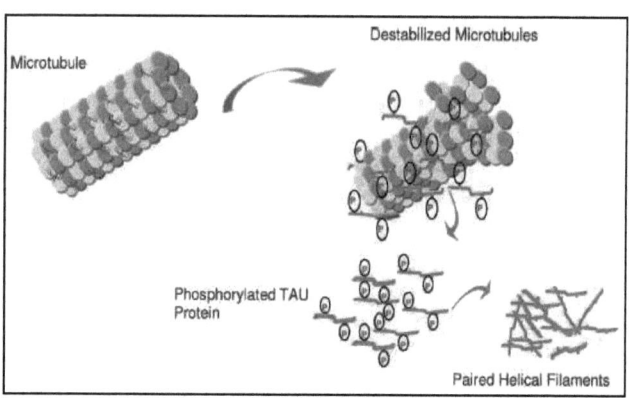

Tau proteins are a group of proteins named as microtubule-associated phosphoproteins that are found in high concentrations in neurons of the central nervous system and are extremely rare in other organs. It has been almost 38 years since tau was discovered as a high temperature resistant and limitedly influenced by acid treatment without loss their function [110, 111].

There is significant evidence that a deviations from normal phosphorylation process (Hyperphosphorylation) results in tau dysfunction and modification of the conformation of tau and decreasing its affinity to microtubules [112].

More studies warranted to stress the role of of tau biomarkers for trial designs and how they may be further eligible for surrogate marker status [113].

Many studies have found CSF biomarkers to be a great tool for AD diagnosis by observing high levels of CSF-T-tau and P-tau, followed by MCI, Stroke and VaD. It is worthy to mention that paradoxical results on CSF biomarkers were found conflicting in VaD (the prototype model of CADASIL) which can be due to possible presence of other underlying pathological alterations [114].

These findings encourage the investigation of P-tau as well as T-tau levels in CADASIL rather than in VaD, since CADASIL reflects a comprehensible pathological model almost exclusively due to cerebrovascular features, making it a clearer model than VaD. Since the levels of P-tau and total tau (T-tau) in the CSF of CADASIL patients were normal, in contrast with elevated values in AD, it's legitimate to consider CADASIL in the differential diagnosis between various neurological diseases.

Conclusion:

The thin discriminating line between AD and VaD remains vague. Therefore, to eliminate this bewilderment and discrepancies in the diagnosis between the AD and VaD, it is worthy to examine a disease that is a microangiopathy and represents VaD with clear milestones and features as is the case of CADASIL. CADASIL is a dominantly inherited mid-adult life disorder causing ischemic strokes, which belongs to vasculopathies and symbolizes a prototype of VaD that provides a unique opportunity for studying its CSF biomarkers and comparing it with CSF biomarkers of AD.

The pathogenesis similarities between CADASIL (a relatively mid-adult disease) with early onset of AD affect the small vessels of the brain suggest plausible molecular mechanisms that are involved in vascular damage and come from the fact that in both diseases genetic mutations occur. CADASIL mutations in NOTCH3 gene generate toxic protein aggregates (Granular Osmiophilic Material- GOM) in the vicinity of vascular smooth muscle cells (VSMCs) causing degeneration and loss of VSMCs in small arteries and arterioles of white matter regions of the brain that lead to dementia, similar to those attributed to mutant forms of the Amyloid Precursor proteins (APP) and presenilins genes who cause overproduction and accumulations of the toxic Aβ42 protein in the brain and collapse of Aβ42 clearance mechanisms in AD. Despite the presumed pathological resemblance, substantial differences between the two phenomena exist especially in the CSF neurochemical phenotypes. These differences in the levels of CSF biomarkers in addition to the neuro-imaging are essential for the differential diagnosis between the two diseases.

The figure 1., below comes to illustrate the dissimilarity of commonly used biomarkers (Aß42, t-tau and P-tau) that are found in the CSF of different neurological diseases such as: AD, VaD, Stroke and CADASIL. Indeed, these divergences are important for the differential diagnosis between the mentioned neurological diseases above. In fact, there is a clear advantage when highlighting the difference in CSF biomarkers between AD and CADASIL that serves to increase the diagnostic accuracy when they used with other biomarkers such as imaging markers.

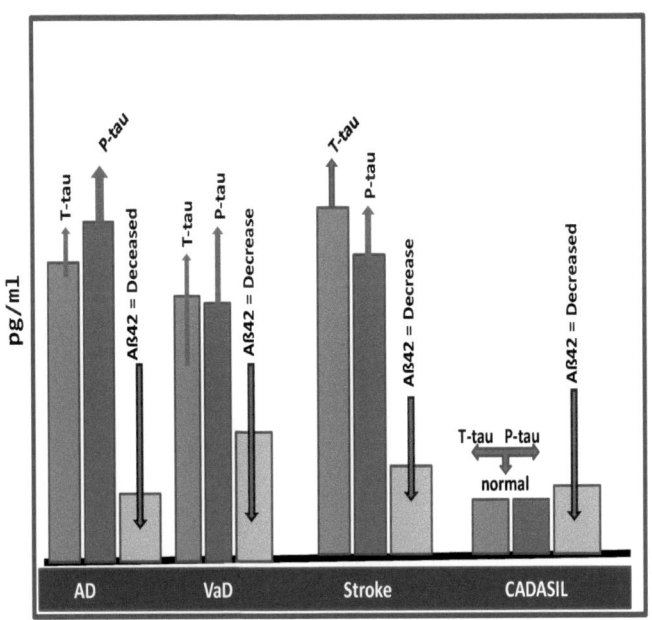

Figure 1. This figure was made according to data from previous studies and from the literature to illustrate the variations in levels of the classical biomarkers (Aß42, t-tau and P-tau), altered generally in the AD, VaD, Stroke and CADASIL. Levels measured by (pg/ml) for all the biomarkers, showed Aß42 with lowest level in AD followed by stroke and moderately decreased in VaD. Total-tau levels are highly increased in stroke followed by AD. Quite the opposite in VaD, studies on these CSF biomarkers showed conflicting results: t-tau levels have been reported to be increased, normal or intermediate, but in any case much lower than in AD. Phosphorylated-tau (P-tau) levels are highly increased in AD followed by stroke but levels of (P-tau) have been reported to be either normal or increased in VaD. In CADASIL total-tau levels and P-tau levels are normal, and Aß42 are markedly deceased and considerably overlapped with AD [23, 115].

References

1. Koffie RM, Hyman BT and Spires-Jones TL (2011) Alzheimer's diseases: synapses gone cold. Molecular Neurodegeneration 6:63. Doi:10.1186/1750-1326-6-63

2. Yassin M, Armaly Z, Bisharat B, Bowirrat A (20-13) Biomarkers for Alzheimer's Disease: Imagination or Reality-View and Review! Journal of Behavioral and Brain Science 3: 393-402.

3. Guerreiro RJ, Gustafson DR, Hardy J (2012) The genetic architecture of Alzheimer's disease: Beyond APP, PSENs AND APOE. Neurobiol Aging 33(3): 437–456.

4. Bowirrat A., Friedland RP., Farrer L., Baldwin C., Korczyn A (2002) Genetic and Environmental Risk factors for Alzheimer's disease in Israeli Arabs. Journal of Molecular Neuroscience 19(1-2):239-245.

5. Alberto Serrano-Pozo, Matthew P. Frosch, Eliezer Masliah, Bradley T. Hyman (2011) Neuropathological Alterations in Alzheimer Disease. Cold Spring Harb Perspect Med 1(1): a006189. doi: 10.1101/cshperspect.a006189 PMCID: PMC3234452.

6. Waldemar G, Dubois B, Emre M (2007) Recommendations for the diagnosis and management of Alzheimer's disease and other disorders associated with dementia: EFNS guideline. *European Journal of Neurology* 14(1):e1–e26.

7. Clifford RJ, Knopman DS, Jagust WJ, Shaw LM, Aisen PS, Weiner MW, Petersen RC, Trojanowski JQ (2010) Hypothetical model of dynamic biomarkers of the Alzheimer's pathological cascade. Lancet Neurol 9(1): 119. doi: 10.1016/S1474-4422(09)70299-6.

8. Jack CR, Holtzman DM (2013) Biomarker modeling of Alzheimer's disease. Neuron 80(6):1347-58.

9. Leszek J, Sochocka M, Gąsiorowski K. Vascular factors and epigenetic modifications in the pathogenesis of Alzheimer's disease (2012) J Neurol Sci 15;323(1-2):25-32. doi: 10.1016/j.jns.2012.09.010. Epub 2012 Sep 29.

10. Pluta R (2004a). Alzheimer lesions after ischemia-reperfusion brain injury. Folia Neuropathol 42:181–186.

11. Pluta R. (2004b). From brain ischemia-reperfusion injury to possible sporadic Alzheimer's disease. Curr Neurovasc Res 1:441-453.

12. Iadecola C (2010) The overlap between neurodegenerative and vascular factors in the pathogenesis of dementia. Acta Neuropathol 120(3): 287–296. doi: 10.1007/s00401-010-0718.

13. Grand Jacob HG, Caspar S, MacDonald Stuart WS (2011) Clinical features and multidisciplinary approaches to dementia care. Journal of Multidisciplinary Healthcare 4 125–147.

14. Iadecola C, Park L, Capone C (2009) Threats to the Mind Aging, Amyloid, and Hypertension. Stroke 40(3 Suppl): S40–S44.

15. Esiri MM, Nagy Z, Smith MZ, Barnetson L, Smith AD (1999) Cerebrovascular disease and threshold for dementia in the early stages of Alzheimer's disease. Lancet 354:919–920.

16. Meng Y, Baldwin CT, Bowirrat A, Inzelberg R, Waraska K, Friedland RP, Farrer LA (2006) Association of Polymorphism in the Angiotensin-converting Enzyme Gene With Alzheimer's Disease in an Israeli-Arab Community. Am J Hum Genet 78:871-877.

17. Schneider JA, Wilson RS, Bienias JL, Evans DA, Bennett DA (2004) Cerebral infarctions and the likelihood of dementia from Alzheimer disease pathology. Neurology 62:1148–1155.

18. Jellinger KA (2013) Pathology and pathogenesis of vascular cognitive impairment—a critical update. Front Aging Neurosci 5: 17.

19. Jellinger KA (2007) The enigma of vascular cognitive disorder and vascular dementia. *Acta Neuropathol* 113(4):349–388.

20. Kalaria RN, Ballard C (1999) Overlap between pathology of Alzheimer disease and vascular dementia. *Alzheimer Disease and Associated Disorders* 13(3):S115–S123.

21. Craggs, L. J.L., Yamamoto, Y., Deramecourt, V. and Kalaria, R. N. (2014) Microvascular Pathology and Morphometrics of Sporadic and Hereditary Small Vessel Diseases of the Brain. Brain Pathology, 24: 495–509. doi: 10.1111/bpa.12177

22. Jellinger KA, Attems J (2010) Prevalence of dementia disorders in the oldest-old: an autopsy study. Acta Neuropathol 119:421–433.

23. Formichi P, Parnetti L, Radi E, Cevenini G, Dotti MT, and Federico A (2010) "CSF Biomarkers Profile in CADASIL—A Model of Pure Vascular Dementia: Usefulness in Differential Diagnosis in the Dementia Disorder," International Journal of Alzheimer's Disease Article Volume 2010, ID 959257, 6 pages. doi:10.4061/2010/959257

24. Roman GC, Tatemichi TK, Erkinjuntti T, Cummings JL, Masdeu JC, Garcia JH, Amaducci L, Orgogozo JM, Brun A, Hofman A, Moody DM, O'Brien MD, Yamaguchi T, Grafman J, Drayer BP, Bennet DP, Fisher M, Ogata J, Kokmen E, Bermejo F, Wolf PA, Gorelick PB, Bick KL, Pajeau AK, Bell MA, DeCarli C, Culebras A, Korczyn AD, Bogousslavsky J, Hartman A, Scheinberg P (1993) Vascular dementia: diagnostic criteria for research studies. Report of the NINDS-AIREN International Workshop. Neurology 43: 250 – 260.

25. Marchesi VT (2014) Alzheimer's disease and CADASIL are heritable, adult-onset dementias that both involve damaged small blood vessels. Cell Mol Life Sci 71(6):949-55. doi: 10.1007/s00018-013-1542-7. Epub 2013 Dec 31.

26. Xinzhen Yin, Dingwen Wu, Jinping Wan, Shenqiang Yan, Min Lou, Guohua Zhao, Baorong Z (2014) Cerebral autosomal dominant arteriopathy with subcortical infarcts and leukoencephalopathy: Phenotypic and mutational spectrum in patients from mainland China. International Journal of Neuroscience 8:1-22.

27. Joutel A, Corpechot C, Ducros A, Vahedi K, Chabriat H, Mouton P, Alamowitch S, Domenga V, Cecillion M, Marechal E, Maciazek J, Vayssiere C, Cruaud C, Cabanis EA, Ruchoux MM, Weissenbach J, Bach JF, Bousser MG, Tournier-Lasserve E (1996) Notch3 mutations in CADASIL, a hereditary adult-onset condition causing stroke and dementia. *Nature* 24:383:707-10.

28. Goebel HH, Meyermann R, Rosin R, Schlote W (1997) Characteristic morphologic manifestation of CADASIL, cerebral autosomal- dominant arteriopathy with subcortical infarcts and leukoencephalopathy, in skeletal muscle and skin. Muscle Nerve 20:625–7.

29. LaPoint SF, Patel U, Rubio A (2000) Cerebral autosomal dominant arteriopathy with subcortical infarcts and leukoencephalopathy (CADASIL). Adv Anat Pathol 7(5):307-21.

30. Malandrini A, Gaudiano C, Gambelli S (2007) Diagnostic value of ultrastructural skin biopsy studies in CADASIL. Neurology 68(17):1430-1432.

31. Bowirrat A (2014) The Pathogenesis of Cerebral Autosomal Dominant Arteriopathy with Subcortical Infarcts and Leukoencephalopathy (CADASIL, OMIM #125310). Ann Clin Cytol Pathol 1(1): 1002.

32. Hampel H, Mitchell A, Blennow K, Frank RA, Brettschneider S, Weller L, Möller HJ (2004) Core biological marker candidates of Alzheimer's disease - perspectives for diagnosis, prediction of outcome and reflection of biological activity. J Neural Transm 111(3): 247–272. doi: 10.1007/s00702-003-0065-z

33. Frangogiannis NG (2012) "Biomarkers: Hopes and Challenges in the Path from Discovery to Clinical Practice," Transla- tional Research 159(4): 197-204. doi:10.1016/j.trsl.2012.01.023.

34. Shaw M, Korecka M, Clark CM, Lee VMY and Trojanowski JQ (2007) "Biomarkers of Neurodegeneration for Diagnosis and Monitoring Therapeutics," Nature Reviews Drug Discovery 6(4): 295-303. doi:10.1038/nrd2176

35. Downing G (2001) "Biomarkers Definitions Working Group. Biomarkers and Surrogate Endpoints," Clinical Pharma- cology & Therapeutics 69; 89-95.

36. Lee J, Devanarayan V, Barrett U, Weiner R, Allinson J, Fountain S, Keller S, Weinryb I, Green M and Duan L (2006) "Fit-for-Purpose Method Development and Validation for Successful Biomarker Measurement," Pharmaceutical Research 23(2): 312-328. doi:10.1007/s11095-005-9045-3

37. Lapraz JC, Hedayat KM, Pauly P (2013) Endobiology: A global approach to systems biology (Part 2 of 2). Glob Adv Health Med 2:32-44.

38. Frank R and Hargreaves R (2003) "Clinical Biomarkers in Drug Discovery and Development," Nature Reviews Drug Dis- covery 2(7): 566-580. doi:10.1038/nrd1130

39. Hess S, Ozoux ML, Gerl M (2011) Biomarker Definition and Validation During Drug Development. Drug discovery and evaluation in clinical pharmacology 1; 223-244.

40. Harald H, Simone L and Khachaturian ZS (2012) "Develop- ment of Biomarkers to Chart All Alzheimer's Disease Stages: The Royal Road to Cutting the Therapeutic Gor- dian Knot," Alzheimer's & Dementia 8(4): 312-336. doi:10.1016/j.jalz.2012.05.2116

41. Dhanasekaran SM (2001) "Delineation of Prognostic Biomar- kers in Prostate Cancer," Nature 412(6849): 822-826. doi:10.1038/35090585

42. Wagner PD, Maruvada P and Srivastava S (2004) "Molecular Diagnostics: A New Frontier in Cancer Prevention," Ex- pert Review of Molecular Diagnostics 4(4): 503-511. doi:10.1586/14737159.4.4.503.

43. Gerde P, Muggenburg BA, Stephens T, Lewis JL, Pyon KH and Dahl AR (1998) "A Relevant Dose of 4-(Me- thylnitrosamino)-1-(3-pyridyl)-1-butanone Is Extensively Metabolized and Rapidly Absorbed in the Canine Tra- cheal Mucosa," Cancer Research 58(7): 1417-1422.

44. Prashanthi V (2010) "Effect of Apolipoprotein E on Biomarkers of Amyloid Load and Neuronal Pathology in Alzheimer Disease," Annals of Neurology 67(3): 308-316.

45. Johnston JA and Hill M (2011) "The Risk and Gamble We Take with Our Patients on Dopamine Agonists," Journal of Neurology, Neurosurgery & Psychiatry 83(3): e1-e1. doi:10.1136/jnnp-2011-301993.155.

46. Golias CH (2005) "Adhesion Molecules in Cancer Invasion and Metastasis," Hippokratia 9(1): 106-114.

47. Kader HA, Tchernev VT, Satyaraj E, Lejnine S, Kotler G, Kingsmore SF and Patel D (2005) "Protein Microar- ray Analysis of Disease Activity in Pediatric Inflamma- tory Bowel Disease Demonstrates Elevated Serum PLGF, IL-7, TGF-β1, and IL-12p40 Levels in Crohn's Disease and Ulcerative Colitis Patients in Remission versus Ac- tive Disease," The American Journal of Gastroenterology 100(2): 414-423. doi:10.1111/j.1572-0241.2005.40819.

48) Carrette O, Demalte I, Scherl A, Yalkinoglu O, Corthals O, Burkhard G and Sanchez JC (2003) "A Panel of Cerebrospinal Fluid Potential Biomarkers for the Diagno- sis of Alzheimer's Disease," Proteomics 3(8): 1486-1494. doi:10.1002/pmic.200300470

49 Weller RO (1998) Pathology of cerebrospinal fluid and interstitial fluid of the CNS: significance for Alzheimer disease, prion disorders and multiple sclerosis.J Neuropathol Exp Neurol 57:885-894.

50. Timo Grimmer, Panagiotis Alexopoulos, Amalia Tsolakidou (2012) "Cerebrospinal Fluid BACE1 Activity and Brain Amyloid Load in Alzheimer's Disease," The Scientific World Journal 1; 1-6. doi:10.1100/2012/712048.

51. Selkoe DJ (1991) "The molecular pathology of Alzheimer's disease." Neuron 6(4): 487-498.

52. Golde TE, Lon SS, Edward HK (2011) "Anti-aβ therapeutics in Alzheimer's disease: the need for a paradigm shift." Neuron 69(2): 203-213.

53. Ibach B, Binder H, Dragon M, Poljansky S, Haen E, Schmitz E and Hajak G (2005) "Cerebrospinal Fluid tau and β- Amyloid in Alzheimer Patients, Disease Controls and an Age-Matched Random Sample," Neurobiology of Aging 27(9):1202-1211.

54. Finder VH, Glockshuber R. (2007) Amyloid-beta aggregation. Neurodegener Dis 4(1):13–27.

55. Hartmann T, Bieger SC, Brühl B, Tienari PJ, Ida N, Allsop D, Roberts GW, Masters CL, Dotti CG, Unsicker K, Beyreuther K (1997) "Distinct sites of intracellular production for Alzheimer's disease A beta40/42 amyloid peptides". Nat Med 3(9): 1016–20. doi:10.1038/nm0997-1016. PMID

56. Allam AR, Kiran KR, Hanuman T (2008) Bioinformatic analysis of Alzheimer's. Disease using functional protein sequences. J Proteomics Bioinform 1: 036–042.

57. Wang R, Wang B, He W, Zheng H (2006) Wild-type presenilin 1 protects against Alzheimer disease mutation-induced amyloid pathology. J Biol Chem 281:15330–15336.

58. Kessels HW, Nguyen LN, Nabavi S, Malinow R (2010) The prion protein as a receptor for amyloid- beta. Nature 466: E3–E4.

59. Tomic JL, Pensalfini A, Head E, Glabe CG (2009) Soluble fibrillar oligomer levels are elevated in Alzheimer's disease brain and correlate with cognitive dysfunction. Neurobiol Dis 35:352–358.

60. Gimbel DA, Nygaard HB, Coffey EE, Gunther EC, Laurén J, Gimbel ZA (2010) Memory impairment in transgenic Alzheimer mice requires cellular prion protein J Neurosci 30: 6367–6374.

61. Zheng H, Koo EH (2011) Biology and pathophysiology of the amyloid precursor protein. Mol Neurodegener 6: 27. doi: 10.1186/1750-1326-6-27

62. Thinakaran G, Koo EH (2008) Amyloid Precursor Protein Trafficking, Processing, and Function. The Journal of Biological Chemistry 283(44):29615-29619. doi:10.1074/jbc.R800019200.

63. Yoo-Hun S, Checler F (2002) "Amyloid precursor protein, presenilins, and α-synuclein: molecular pathogenesis and pharmacological applications in Alzheimer's disease." Pharmacological reviews 54(3) 469-525.

64. Soriano S (2001) "The amyloidogenic pathway of amyloid precursor protein (APP) is independent of its cleavage by caspases." The Journal of biological chemistry 276(31): 29045-29050.

65. Yang M, Virassamy B, Vijayaraj SL, Lim Y, Saadipour K, Wang YJ (2013) The intracellular domain of sortilin interacts with amyloid precursor protein and regulates its lysosomal and lipid raft trafficking. PLoS ONE 8(5): e63049

66. Simons M (1998) "Cholesterol depletion inhibits the generation of β-amyloid in hippocampal neurons." Proceedings of the National Academy of Sciences 95.11: 6460-6464.

67. Butler D, Bahr BA (2006) "Oxidative Stress and Lyso- somes: CNS-Related Consequences and Implications for Lysosomal Enhancement Strategies and Induction of Autophagy," Antioxidants & Redox Signaling 8(1-2): 185-196.

68. Avila J, Lucas JJ, Perez M, Hernandez F (2004) Role of tau protein in both physiological and pathological conditions. Physiol Rev 84: 361–384.

69. Graff-Radford NR, Crook JE, Lucas J, Boeve BF, Knopman DS, Ivnik RJ and Younkin SG (2007) "Associa- tion of Low Plasma Abeta42/Abeta40 Ratios with In- creased Imminent Risk for Mild Cognitive Impairment and Alzheimer Disease," Archives of Neurology 64(3): 354. doi:10.1001/archneur.64.3.354

70. Blennow K, Vanmechelen E and Hampel H (2001) "CSF To- tal tau, Ab42 and Phosphorylated tau Protein as Bio- markers for Alzheimer's Disease" Molecular Neurobiol- ogy 24(1-3): 87-97.

71. Fagan AM, Mintun MA, Mach RH, Lee SY, Dence CS, Shah AR, LaRossa GN, Spinner ML, Klunk WE, Mathis CA, DeKosky ST, Morris JC Holtzman DM (2006) "Inverse Relation between *in Vivo* Amy- loid Imaging Load and Cerebrospinal Fluid Abeta42 in Humans," Annals of Neurology 59(3): 512-519. doi:10.1002/ana.20730

72. Schneider, Lon, Richard Kennedy, and Gary Cutter. "Amnestic MCI/prodromal Alzheimer's disease with more severe memory deficit is indistinguishable from diagnosed Alzheimer disease: Implications for the validity of clinical trials and biomarkers." *Alzheimer's & Dementia* 7.4 (2011): S681-S682.

73. Ju Yo-El S, Lucey BP, Holtzman DM (2014) Sleep and Alzheimer disease pathology—a bidirectional relationship. Nature Reviews Neurology 10; 115–119.

74. Fagan AM, Roe CM, Xiong C, Mintun MA, Morris JC and Holtzman DM (2007) "Cerebrospinal Fluid tau/ beta-Amyloid(42) Ratio as a Prediction of Cognitive De- cline in Nondemented Older Adults," Archives of Neu- rology 64(3): 343-349. doi:10.1001/archneur.64.3.noc60123

75. Sjögren M, Davidsson P and Aallin A (2002) "Decreased CSF β-Amyloid42 in Alzheimer's Disease and Amyotrophic Lateral Sclerosis May Reflect Mismetabolism of β- Amyloid Induced by separate mechanisms," Dementia and Geriatric Cognitive Disorders 13: 112-118. doi:10.1159/000048642.

76. Strozyk D, Blennow K, White LR and Launer LJ (2003) "CSF Aβ42 Levels Correlate with Amyloid-Neuropatho- logy in a Population-Based Autopsy Study," Neurology 60(4): 652-656. doi:10.1212/01.WNL.0000046581.81650.D0

77. Hachinski VC, Bowler JV (1993) Vascular dementia. Neurology 43:2159–2160.

78. Chui HC, Victoroff JI, Margolin D (1992) Criteria for the diagnosis of ischemic vascular dementia proposed by the State of California Alzheimer's Disease Diagnostic and Treatment Centers. Neurology 42:473–480

79. Jellinger KA (2008) Morphologic diagnosis of "vascular dementia"—a critical update. J Neurol Sci 270:1–12.

80. Erkinjuntti T, Gauthier S (2009) The concept of vascular cognitive impairment. Front Neurol Neurosci 24:79–85.

81. Breteler MM (2000) Vascular risk factors for Alzheimer's disease: an epidemiologic perspective. Neurobiol Aging 21:153–160.

82. Iadecola C, Gorelick PB (2003) Converging pathogenic mechanisms in vascular and neurodegenerative dementia. Stroke 34:335–337.

83. Kalaria RN (2000) The role of cerebral ischemia in Alzheimer's disease. Neurobiol Aging 21:321–330.

84. Nagy Z, Esiri MM, Jobst KA (1997) The effects of additional pathology on the cognitive deficit in Alzheimer disease. J Neuropathol Exp Neurol 56:165–170.

85. Snowdon DA, Greiner LH, Mortimer JA (1997) Brain infarction and the clinical expression of Alzheimer disease. The Nun Study. JAMA 277:813–817.

86. Iadecola C (2004) Neurovascular regulation in the normal brain and in Alzheimer's disease. Nat Rev Neurosci 5:347–360.

87. Jiong S (2000) "Vascular abnormalities: the insidious pathogenesis of Alzheimer's disease." Neurobiology of aging 21(2). 357-361.

88. Koike MA, Green KN, Blurton-Jones M, LaFerla FM (2010) Oligemic hypoperfusion differentially affects tau and amyloid-{beta} Am J Pathol 177(1): 300-310. doi: 10.2353/ajpath.2010.090750. [PMC free article] [PubMed]

89. Li L, Zhang X, Yang D (2009) Hypoxia increases Abeta generation by altering beta- and gamma-cleavage of APP. Neurobiol Aging 30:1091–1098. [PubMed]

90. Tesco G, Koh YH, Kang EL (2007) Depletion of GGA3 stabilizes BACE and enhances beta-secretase activity. Neuron 54:721–737. [PMC free article] [PubMed

91. Cirrito JR, Yamada KA, Finn MB (2005) Synaptic activity regulates interstitial fluid amyloid-beta levels in vivo. Neuron 48:913–922. [PubMed

92. Deane R, Wu Z, Sagare A (2004) LRP/amyloid beta-peptide interaction mediates differential brain efflux of Abeta isoforms. Neuron 43:333–344. [PubMed]

93 Kapaki E (2001) "Highly increased CSF tau protein and decreased β-amyloid (1–42) in sporadic CJD: a discrimination from Alzheimer's disease?." Journal of Neurology, Neurosurgery & Psychiatry 71(3): 401-403.

94. Anders W, Sjögren M (2001) "Cerebrospinal fluid cytoskeleton proteins in patients with subcortical white-matter dementia." Mechanisms of ageing and development 122(16); 1937-1949.

95. Welge V, Fiege O, Lewczuk P, Mollenhauer B, Esselmann H, Klafki HW, Bibl M (2009) Combined CSF tau, p-tau181 and amyloid-β 38/40/42 for diagnosing Alzheimer's disease. Journal of neural transmission 116(2), 203-212.

96. Pfefferkorn T, von Stuckrad-Barre S, Herzog J, Gasser T, Hamann GF, Dichgans M (2001). Reduced cerebrovascular CO(2) reactivity in CADASIL: a transcranial Doppler sonography study. Stroke 32: 17–21.

97. Paul TJ, Hardy J, Fischbeck HK (2002) "Toxic proteins in neurodegenerative disease." Science 296(5575):1991-1995.

98. Morris M, Maeda S, Vossel K and Mucke L (2011) "The Many Faces of Tau," Neuron 70(3): 410-426. doi:10.1016/j.neuron.2011.04.009

99. Buée L, Bussiere T, Buee-Scherrer V, Delacourte A and Hof PR (2000) "Tau Protein Isoforms, Phosphorylation and Role in Neurodegenerative Disorders," Brain Re- search Reviews 33(1): 95-130. doi:10.1016/S0165-0173(00)00019-9

100. Feijoo C, Campbell DG, Jakes R, Goedert M and Cuenda A (2005) "Evidence That Phosphorylation of the Micro- tubule-Associated Protein Tau by SAPK4/p38δ at Thr50 Promotes Microtubule Assembly," Journal of Cell Sci- ence 118(2): 397-408. doi:10.1242/jcs.01655

101. Boekhoorn K, Terwel D, Biemans B, Borghgraef P, Wiegert O, Ramakers GJ and Lucassen PL (2006) "Improved Long-Term Potentiation and Memory in Young tau- P301L Transgenic Mice before Onset of Hyperphos- phorylation and Tauopathy. J Neurosci 26(13): 3514-3523.

102. Vandermeeren M, Mercken M and Vanmechelen E (1993) "Detection of τ Proteins in Normal and Alzheimer's Dis- ease Cerebrospinal Fluid with a Sensitive Sandwich En- zyme-Linked Immunosorbent Assay. Journal of Neuro- chemistry 61: 1828-1834. doi:10.1111/j.1471-4159.1993.tb09823.

103. Hansson O, Zetterberg H, Buchhave P, Londos E, Blennow K and Minthon L (2006) "Association between CSF Biomarkers and Incipient Alzheimer's Disease in Patients with Mild Cognitive Impairment: A Follow-Up Study. The Lancet Neurology 5(3): 228-234. doi:10.1016/S1474-4422(06)70355-6

104. Carrette O, Demalte I, Scherl A, Yalkinoglu O, Corthals O, Burkhard G and Sanchez JC (2003) "A Panel of Cerebrospinal Fluid Potential Biomarkers for the Diagno- sis of Alzheimer's Disease. Proteomics 3(8): 1486-1494. doi:10.1002/pmic.200300470

105. Lanari A and Parnetti L (2009) "Cerebrospinal Fluid Bio- markers and Prediction of Conversion in Patients with Mild Cognitive Impairment: 4-Year Follow-Up in a Rou- tine Clinical Setting. The Scientific World Journal 9: 961-966. doi:10.1100/tsw.2009.106

106. Mattsson N, Zetterberg H, Hansson O, Andreasen N, Parnetti L, Jonsson M and Blennow K (2009) "CSF Biomarkers and Incipient Alzheimer Disease in Patients with Mild Cognitive Impairment," The Journal of the American Medical Association 302(4): 385-393. doi:10.1001/jama.2009.1064

107. Zanusso G, Fiorini M, Righetti PG and Monaco S (2011) "Specific and Surrogate Cerebrospinal Fluid Markers in Creutzfeldt—Jakob Disease," Advances in Neurobiology 2: 455-467.

108. Formichi P, Parnetti L, Radi E, Cevenini G, Dotti MT, Federico A (2008) "CSF Levels of β-Amyloid 1-42, Tau and Phosphorylated Tau Protein in CADASIL," European Journal of Neurology 15(11): 1252-1255. doi:10.1111/j.1468-1331.2008.02277.

109. Stanford PA, Halliday GM, Brooks WS, Kwok JB, Storey CE, Creasey H, Schofield PR (2011) "Progressive Supranuclear Palsy Pathology Caused by a Novel Silent Mutation in Exon 10 of the *Tau* Gene Ex- pansion of the Disease Phenotype Caused by *Tau* Gene Mutations," Brain 123(5): 880-893.

110. Cleveland DW, Hwo SY and Kirschner MW (1977) "Physical and Chemical Properties of Purified *Tau* Factor and the Role of *Tau* in Microtubule Assembly," Journal of Molecular Biology 116(2): 227- 247.

111. Morris M, Maeda S, Vossel K and Mucke L (2011) "The Many Faces of Tau," Neuron 70(3): 410-426. doi:10.1016/j.neuron.2011.04.009

112. Buée L, Bussiere T, Buee-Scherrer V, Delacourte A and Hof PR (2000) "Tau Protein Isoforms, Phosphorylation and Role in Neurodegenerative Disorders," Brain Re- search Reviews 33(1): 95-130.

113. Hampel H, Blennow K, Shaw LM, Hoessler YC, Zetterberg H and Trojanowski JQ (2009) "Total and Phosphory- lated *Tau* Protein as Biological Markers of Alzheimer's Disease," Experimental Gerontology 45(1): 30-40. doi:10.1016/j.exger.2009.10.010

114. Stenset V, Johnsen L, Kocot D (2006) Associations between white matter lesions, cerebrovascular risk factors, and low CSF Aβ42. *Neurology* 67(5):830–833. [PubMed]

115. Kaerst L, Kuhlmann A, Wedekind D, Stoeck K, Lange P, Zerr I (2013) Cerebrospinal fluid biomarkers in Alzheimer's disease, vascular dementia and ischemic stroke patients: a critical analysis. J Neurol 260(11):2722-7. doi: 10.1007/s00415-013-7047-3.

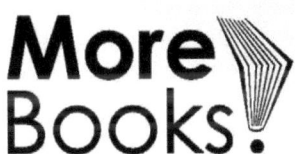
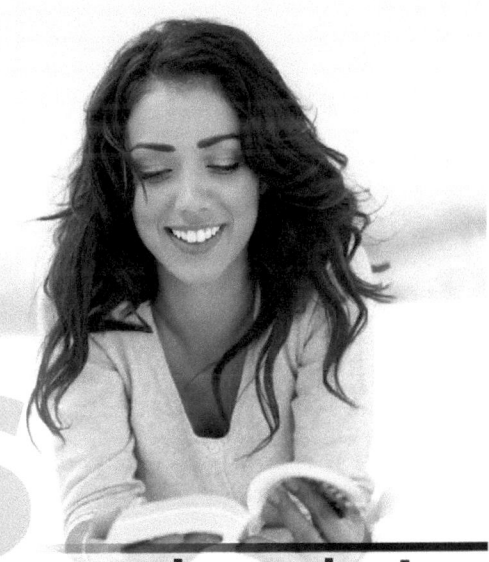
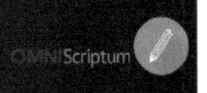

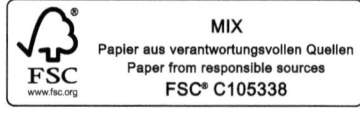